Saying Good-Bye to Managed Care

Building Your Independent Psychotherapy Practice

D1256416

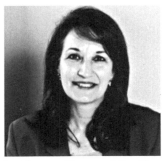

Sandra Haber, PhD, a fellow of the American Psychological Association, was honored as Distinguished Psychologist of the Year in 1993–4. Her full-time affiliation is as a private practitioner in New York City.

Dr. Haber is the editor of *Breast Cancer: A Psychological Treatment Manual* (Springer, 1995) and co-author of *Men, Women and Prostate Cancer: A Medical and Psychological Guide for Women and the Men They Love* (2000). In 1999, she was given the Blue Ribbon Education Award by Cancer Care and the Naussau County Psychological Association. Dr. Haber is the Past President of the Division of Independent Practice of the American Psychological Association.

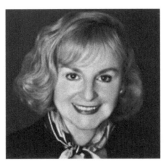

Elaine Rodino, PhD, has been an independent practitioner for more than 20 years and is currently in full-time private practice in Santa Monica, California. Her work has focused on individuals and couples dealing with a variety of life issues including career matters, divorce, anxiety, and depression.

She is a past-president of Los Angeles County Psychological Association and is current representative from Los Angeles to the Board of the California Psychological Association. She is also a member of the American Psychological Association's Division of Psychotherapy, and Division for the Study of Men and Masculinity. She was named a fellow of the Los Angeles Society of Clinical Psychologists, elected to the National Academies of Practice and received the Karl F. Heiser APA Award for Federal Advocacy in Psychology.

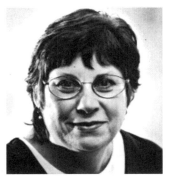

Iris Lipner, CSW, is a Board Certified Diplomate in Clinical Social Work in the private practice of psychotherapy and psychoanalysis in New York City. She works with adults, specializing in women's issues and clients with chronic illness; and with couples. Ms. Lipner serves as a consultant to professionals building an independent practice and has recently taught a workshop, "Social Worker-Psychotherapist: Creating an Independent Practice," in the NYC Chapter of National Association of Social Workers, 2000 Continuing Education program. She has a Certificate in Psychoanalysis from the Manhattan Institute for Psychoanalysis; is a Founding Member and serves on the Board of the American Mental Health Alliance-New York; is a Fellow, New York State Society for Clinical Social Work; and a Diplomate in Clinical Social Work, National Association of Social Workers.

Saying Good-Bye to Managed Care

Building Your Independent Psychotherapy Practice

Sandra Haber, PhD, **Elaine Rodino,** PhD
and **Iris Lipner,** CSW

 Springer Publishing Company

Springer Publishing Company, Inc.
536 Broadway
New York, NY 10012-3955

Acquisitions Editor: Bill Tucker
Production Editor: Pamela Lankas
Cover design by Susan Hauley

01 02 03 04 05 / 5 4 3 2 1

Library of Congress Cataloging-in-Publication Data

Haber, Sandra.
    Saying good-bye to managed care : building your independent
    psychotherapy practice / Sandra Haber, Elaine Rodino, and
    Iris Lipner, authors.
        p. cm.
    Includes bibliographical references and index.
    ISBN 0-8261-1383-4
    1. Psychotherapy—Practice—United States.   2. Mental health
services—United States—Marketing.   I. Rodino, Elaine. II. Lipner,
Iris. III. Title.

    RC465.6 .H42 2000
    616.89'14'068—dc21

                                   00-063527

Contents

Part IV   Basic Tools of the Trade

Part V   Intermediate Tools of the Trade

Part VI   Advanced Tools of the Trade

Part VII   Putting It All Together

Foreword

Somewhere in the 1990s, the phrase "independent practice" became a painful oxymoron. The managed care industry was succeeding in its effort to take control over professional practice and bring independent practice to an end.

Each of us who has decided not to work under the managed care system has had her or his own reasons. Mine had to do with values, excellence, and meaningful work; with being free to do good in the world and easing some of the pain I saw in my clients; and with the freedom to choose the influences over me. It had to do with a need for independence, dignity, and integrity. To a lesser degree but still important, my decision also had to do with wanting a reasonable, professional fee for my work.

By September of 1991, having been licensed for a little over a year and seeing my new private practice start to grow, I finally felt in control of my own life. Striving for excellence, I had just begun my psychoanalytic training and looked forward to the rest of my professional life.

Then, in November of 1991, the teachers I was treating began to tell me that their insurance was changing. Their copayment had been about $60/week, a sum that they felt was reasonable and affordable. Their new plan promised "better benefits at lower cost" and their copayment would be only $15. But I needed to be accepted into "the plan." What? I had to be accepted by some corporation to continue working with these patients?

I resisted signing up and my patients began getting angry with me. The more I learned about the plan and managed care, the more outraged I felt. Outrage became fear and depression. I discovered that my colleagues were also having similar experiences.

My sensitivity to issues of interpersonal and political power led me to re-read George Orwell's *1984* and Aldous Huxley's *Brave New World* as well as a few of Erich Fromm's books (e.g., *The Sane Society, Man For Himself, Escape From Freedom, The Heart of Man,* and *The*

Anatomy of Human Destructiveness). I recommend these books to anyone interested in the deeper implications of the "industrialization" of health care.

These books validated the sense of control and malevolence I perceived in managed care. I better understood the purpose of managed care's "Newspeak" in which we "providers" were to work in "behavioral health," not in mental health, psychology, psychiatry, social work, or counseling. A patient's "functioning" would determine his or her need for treatment and we would ask case managers for authorization to administer appropriate techniques during an "episode" of treatment.

Language was created to narrow the range of thought and change how we saw ourselves, our patients, and our roles. Euphemisms and slogans were created to make destructive and abusive things look beneficial or benign. While colleagues argued that we should simply explain to corporate executives what patients really need, I knew that managed care was about money, not people, and that therapists who did not conform to the Party dictates would be banished to professional Siberia.

I knew that managed care was about control and profit. It was about forcing a humanistic treatment into a sterile, mechanical, industrial model for the sake of corporate profit. It was about being forced into an economic dependency on people who had only contempt for our patients and our profession. It was about having to betray my patients' privacy and confidentiality in order to beg for permission to provide a handful of sessions at a time. It was about patients losing control of their own therapy. I knew, too, that the industry would create training programs to ensure that new clinicians knew only "managed techniques" and nothing of psychodynamics or longer term therapies. This was a new form of indentured servitude, but with no release after 7 years. (For those interested in articles by Dr. Shore that expand on these ideas, please call 1-888-SAY-NO-MC or see www.nomanagedcare.org). The demoralization was deep and pervasive among professionals.

In November 1992, a few colleagues and I founded the National Coalition of Mental Health Professionals and Consumers with the goals of exposing, regulating, and ultimately replacing managed care. But despite my activism, despite knowing how destructive managed care was going to be, and despite the fact that I wanted no part of it, I was still a fairly new clinician and my fear that I could not support myself without managed care led me to join a couple of plans in 1993.

I felt horrible each time I had to write or phone in a report on my patients. I felt I was betraying their privacy. Like other therapists, I now had extra hours of unpaid paperwork.

There were two "final straws" for me. One was when one of my patients needed a psychiatrist on her plan. Though I knew good psychiatrists, none were on her list. Having been abused by a previous psychiatrist, her fear was so overwhelming that she needed nine sessions just to prepare emotionally for her first visit to this unknown psychiatrist. The second was when I realized that the fear of not staying in the insurance companies' good graces had influenced my professional judgment. Trained to question patients who want to quit therapy at times that surprise me, I did not challenge one young woman when she said she thought it was time to "try it on her own." I doubted my training. Maybe I do see people too long; maybe I do see their deficits more than their strengths. So, I didn't challenge her. About a year later, she came back very depressed, tearful, and filled with guilt. She told me she had lied to me when she said she thought she was ready to stop therapy. In reality, she wanted to do something she knew I would try to convince her not to do. Though I rarely tell people what to do, in this instance, she was right. The insidious nature of this industry hit me with tremendous impact. I knew I could not continue to work under this system.

The only solution for my patients' well-being and my own was to get out of managed care. This was frightening, but I could not tolerate this demoralizing experience nor allow it to control me, my work, and my patients. My income dropped by one third within a few months and took quite some time to build it back up.

I could have used this book back then. Sandra Haber, Elaine Rodino, and Iris Lipner have written *Saying Good-Bye to Managed Care* to help people who want independence from this demeaning, destructive, and demoralizing system. Whether you want to keep your practice limited to psychotherapy or are open to expanding into related areas, Haber, Rodino, and Lipner have written this book to tell you that you can survive without managed care and can do well, and they will help you do both. They have provided a wealth of questions and ideas that can stimulate your thinking and turn it into action so you can create your own truly independent practice and work in a way that is in synch with your values and with who you are as a person.

One request, though, as you achieve your independence from managed care: Please become or remain supportive of political action against this industry. Remember that there are people with too little money to pay for good therapy out-of-pocket. Remember that we are all "consumers" of health care and so are all those we love. Find your personal solution for your practice, but help solve the larger problem, too. We must all continue working to defeat this industry and bring about a better system.

Until managed care is gone, though, "independent practice" does not have to be a contradiction in terms. There is life outside of managed care. And it is far better than life inside managed care.

KAREN SHORE, PHD

Karen Shore, PhD, has a truly independent practice in Westbury, NY. She is also co-founder and President of the National Coalition of Mental Health Professionals and Consumers, Inc.

Acknowledgments

To change is to be challenged. Rising to the challenges of managed care and building an independent psychotherapy practice is most easily accomplished in an environment of support and affirmation. Our experience in writing and researching the materials for this book was facilitated in a similar manner. We thank our partners and spouses, Ron Dannenberg, Bob Rodino, and Tim Platt for providing unwavering enthusiasm and encouragement for this project. We also thank our professional colleagues for so generously sharing their experiences and strategies for business success. Our outside readers, psychologist Dennis Steele and soon-to-be psychologist Rachel McClements provided invaluable feedback on earlier versions of this manuscript. We also thank you, the reader, for having the faith to use our book as a guide to build your successful independent psychotherapy practice.

Part I

Can I Run My Practice Without Managed Care?

Chapter 1

Saying Goodbye to Managed Care: How You Can Do It

In the middle of difficulty lies opportunity.
—Albert Einstein

The systematic growth of managed care has unpredictably challenged the independent practice of psychotherapy, simultaneously threatening our professionalism, livelihood, and ethics. Many refer to this threat as a crisis in health care because it effects the way in which psychotherapeutic services are provided and who provides them.

The Chinese symbol for crisis serves as an apt metaphor; it is a configuration of two characters: one representing difficulty, the other opportunity. The aspect of crisis representing difficulty reminds us of the numerous obstacles and threats facing our profession. The aspect of crisis representing opportunity reminds us that even during these difficult times a successful psychotherapy practice is possible through wise decision making and strategic planning. By focusing on opportunity, the problems of managed care can be minimized and alternative paths can be developed that preserve professional integrity and ethical principles while providing attractive financial compensation.

SOME THOUGHTS ABOUT YOU, OUR READER

We know that you, our readers, are well educated and well trained. You have honed your skills with postgraduate supervised experience and see yourself as a professional, competent, and skilled psychotherapist.

3

The joy of the psychotherapy work you do is based on the help you give to others. Daily feelings of success have been your rewards as you participate in the changes that evolve in your patients. You see your patients taking positive steps and productive risks and becoming self-confident and self-reliant.

Recently, you have seen managed care have an impact on your work, erode your joy, limit your patients' success and destroy your financial autonomy. You are concerned about your own ability to manage these obstacles although your intuitive self suspects that you have all the abilities you need to surmount this problem. Your inner voice is right. Dealing with managed care requires exactly the same skills you have used many times before. Think back to the various hurdles you have faced in life. Perhaps they were in academic course work, with difficult supervisors or unmanageable patients. Perhaps there were financial hardships, family dysfunction, or medical illness. Rarely does the personal or professional course of life run smoothly.

In each case, the obstacle you faced could have stopped you but it did not. In fact, conquering the obstacle made you stronger, increased your self-esteem, and contributed to your effectiveness as an empathetic therapist. Remembering these challenges and your mastery of them will help give you the strength and resolve your need to build an independent psychotherapy practice.

As you make the transition to an independent psychotherapy practice, remember that in your work as a psychotherapist, you ask your patients to "have faith" and reach beyond their ordinary range of beliefs and behaviors. Each session you help them inch forward towards their goal. You know their task will be arduous, methodical and difficult. They will experience doubt and uncertainty. If they persevere, they will succeed.

All difficult changes require this leap of faith. But as progress occurs and achievements and victories increase, the processes of change becomes easier . As you face the challenges of managed care, you need ask of yourself the same leap of faith that you ask of your patients—no more, no less.

You are now faced with a series of new challenges. In addition to matters related to privacy, ethics, confidentiality, and professionalism, there is still one final professional issue left to discuss: managed care's low fees and frequent nonreimbursement tactics. Together, this deluge of troubles forces us to face the reality that not only can you not deliver the psychotherapy care appropriate for your patient, but also you will not even be paid your contracted fee.

For many of us, these "managed care blues" will be the final straw that move us toward an independent psychotherapy practice. As you read each scenario, make use of your frustration as a business fuel that moves you toward a thriving private practice.

Situation 1. Treatment is going along just fine and then there is a delay in reauthorization. Either you forgot to send in the form on time or you filled it out incorrectly, but in any case the next session is not covered.

Situation 2. You notice from the managed care reimbursement that some sessions were left unpaid for the wrong reason or omitted for no reason. You call the company and go over the dates of treatment with a representative, and he agrees that this was an "error." This begins to happen more and more frequently.

Situation 3. Your sessions are authorized, but you notice that several months go by before you receive reimbursement. You wind up using your savings or credit line to bridge your expenses between payments from the managed care company.

Situation 4. The patient is ill or acting out and cancels the session. The managed care company will not cover missed sessions. You attempt to collect directly from the patient, but she is not used to paying when she does receive services, much less when she does not. The fee for the session remains uncollected.

Situation 5. You routinely fill out lengthy treatment reports, call the managed care company, and remain on hold for at least 30 minutes, spending time correcting its errors or complying with its latest regulation. You are not compensated for any of this time.

Situation 6. You receive a new referral who can pay your usual and customary fee and then find out that the client is covered by a managed care organization (MCO) for which you are considered a "provider." You are then obligated to change the financial arrangement and wind up with a reduced fee.

Situation 7. There is an emergency situation, and the patient needs to be seen more than one time that week. The managed care company will not cover this. Your choice is to abandon the patient or to deliver what will probably be a pro bono hour.

Situation 8. The client's hours of work change and she or he needs a prime time hour. Your dilemma is to grant the prime time hour and forego potential private pay income or to abandon the client.

Situation 9. The "MCO clinical team" has telephonic treatment plan reviews. You need to spend time preparing for this review and then spend the time on the phone discussing the case. You probably will not be given authorization for additional sessions, and you realize that you have wasted hours doing this.

Situation 10. Your client's benefit coverage changes. She or he now has a new managed care company that you did not know about until you not receive payment from the old MCO. You are required to join the new network in order to get paid and back bill when and if you are accepted. If you are not accepted, you will need to persuade your client to pay for these services or you are out the money.

Situation 11. You thought you did a great job and got your treatment plans in on time, used the correct diagnostic codes, and filled out all their forms appropriately. To your surprise you get a note that you have two sessions to terminate psychotherapy treatment because the MCO does not think your client's personality disorder falls under the rubric of "medical necessity."

We hope you are completely fed up and ready to make a change. None of us signed up for this. It is clear that a direct-pay, primarily managed care–free private psychotherapy practice provides a win–win for all involved. Patients win because they receive quality care in a confidential environment. Professionals win because they are able to earn a living and maintain their self-respect.

HOW THIS BOOK WILL HELP

Developing your direct-pay practice—be it in addition to or instead of managed care—takes work, courage, creativity, and stamina. This book concentrates on boosting your natural responses and abilities, stimulating your creativity, and reminding you of your long-forgotten strengths. We will shepherd and encourage you on this journey. You will not be alone. We start by reminding you of the work you love and arousing the healthy anger and outrage at the problems the managed care crisis has created. These feelings are needed to energize you in your movement toward an independent psychotherapy practice. They are your fuel.

Next, we will have a long, honest, and serious talk about money and face the fact that goodness and caring aside, money matters if you are operating a business—and an independent psychotherapy practice is a business. After our discussion of money, we will help you to recognize your strengths and build on them in slow manageable increments to reshape your practice. We suggest ways to sharpen your skills and to add some "people appeal" to your psychotherapy vocabulary. Our marketing tools will give you the graduate education you never had but always wanted. We have graded our chapters on marketing tools from basic to advanced so that you can choose a marketing effort that feels right for you and is congruent with the time and energy you are able to invest. You may choose to jazz up traditional tools, such as stationery and business cards, or move into the world of e-commerce and virtual groups. We provide the how to—you decide what is right for you.

Finally, we provide an example of a complete, marketable psychotherapy practice that includes all of the marketing materials you need for a successful independent psychotherapy practice. You can copy or adapt these materials as you desire.

- Think of this book as the course you never had in graduate school. Your education probably did not include business management, referral opportunities, or networking skills. This book is a course in how to create a solid referral base and be a psychotherapist-businessperson.
- Think of this book as a personal mentor with the wisdom to outline the steps, explain the various solutions, and help you find the best fit for your unique talents and abilities. It will pace you so you avoid burnout; it will urge you on when you delay.
- Think of this book as a support system, a chorus of voices and experience from seasoned psychotherapists who have successfully traveled this route.
- Think of this book as a personal coach who will encourage, support, and challenge you in your mission.
- Think of this book as a graphic artist with specific suggestions and examples of customized marketing tools.
- Think of this book as a public relations agency with model press releases and pitch letters you can customize for your own practice.

Throughout the book you will notice that our recommended methods do not involve any major retraining or new training. We have focused on repackaging and supplementing what you already know so you can successfully sell your services to a direct pay market.

We believe that ultimately ending your relationship with managed care is like many of life's good-byes. It is a process during which you can achieve a sense of mastery, and one that can feel natural and right. It is a process that can make you stronger rather than weaker, wealthier rather than poorer, and honored rather than sorrowful. The crisis of managed care presents us with an unprecedented opportunity to challenge our abilities, demonstrate our strengths, and enhance our personal power through the pride and satisfaction of mastery. Most important, by the end of this book, you will know that if and when you choose, you too will be able to join us in saying good-bye to managed care.

Chapter 2

Are You a New Professional or Graduate Student or Are You New to Private-Pay Practice?

I f you are a graduate student, new professional or are thinking of leaving your clinic, hospital position, or MCO panel, you may find yourself unpreprepared and unnerved at the prospect of developing a private pay psychotherapy practice. No matter when you attended graduate school, your courses probably included research methods, statistics and personality theories. If your program was more cutting edge or if you are a more recent graduate, you may have been exposed to the emerging areas of practice in which mental health professionals will be needed, such as business consulting, health psychology, or forensics. We bet, however, that you did not have a single course in practice building, marketing, or business operations. Students leave their graduate programs well-educated and well-trained but bewildered about applying their skills to a private-pay market.

Beginning a private practice is an overwhelming experience and one with which each psychotherapist needs to come to terms. Most likely you have never been taught how to develop an independent practice or how to nurture your practice to grow. Perhaps your training has been flooded with nay-saying comments. For example, graduate students and new graduates are sometimes warned by their professors that they had better not think of opening a practice in a large metropolitan area. The theory is that the market is filled and that the only successful locations left for independent practice are in rural areas. This misguided advice has been given for many, many years. We find it to be entirely without substance. In fact, metropolitan areas typically breed educated consumers who are more accepting and interested in psychotherapy when compared with their rural counterparts. A high density of psychotherapists also means that there will be easy and convenient access for consumers, encouraging routine therapy appointments that can be incorporated into hectic schedules. In addition, busy urban areas contribute to the anonymity of treatment that patients typically find comforting. Finally, a plethora of therapists means that there will be a wide choice of therapeutic specialties and delivery styles that can accommodate individual needs and preferences. Therefore, we believe that you can make your practice wherever you would like it to be. Whether you prefer to live in a city, the suburbs, or a rural area, you can successfully begin and nurture your private-pay practice.

On the other hand, a true, but little discussed, impediment to private practice that affects graduate students and new professionals is the impact that managed care has had on the curriculum in many graduate departments and schools. Less emphasis is placed on more traditional forms of treatment and evaluations; more courses and training are concerned with how to write treatment plans for managed care reviewers. More schools teach their graduates to be ready for the managed care marketplace rather than to be healers of people in emotional distress. In other words, graduate school educators have interpreted today's managed care situation to be a major change in how psychotherapy is understood and conducted. We believe that this is a serious misinterpretation. Managed care is only a change in how to pay for psychotherapy. Managed care is about business, not about treatment of people and their needs. In theory then, there should be no change in teaching how to practice good psychotherapy. This is a critical point to consider. If you want to develop an independent psychotherapy practice, you will need to provide a service that offers excellent care.

As a professional new to a private-pay practice, one of the most frightening concerns is that of autonomy and responsibility. To address this concern, we recommend continuing supervision with either a respected senior mentor or a peer supervision consulting group. Those of you with considerable hospital, clinic, or managed care experience may be surprised at this recommendation. However, we have found that institutional work experiences do not necessarily contribute to private practice building skills. Rather, because each of these experiences involves managed care, there is often a tight regimen of prescribed treatment plans with specific interventions delivered within a set number of treatment sessions. This can typically create a quick, though often temporary, solution that gives the patient, the psychotherapist, and the supervisor a sense of satisfaction. Additionally, most or all of the fee in each of these settings is covered by a third party, so money issues are usually not addressed.

We believe that to develop an ongoing private-pay practice, you need to be able to use different treatment modalities and to provide long-term care to patients who warrant it. Psychotherapist Karen Shore[1] notes that her supervisees have not been trained in delivering psychotherapy beyond the typical 20-session allotment. They are not familiar, nor comfortable, with an ongoing therapeutic patient-therapist relationship. This limitation means that the psychotherapist will be unable to provide the long-term therapy needed to facilitate changes in character that many patients require. Additionally, third-party payment is often not available in a private pay situation; it is necessary for the therapist and the patient to deal directly with the issue of fees.

The successful development of a private practice comes from mastery of information, the development of short- and long-term therapeutic skills, and the ability to function as a businessperson. This can be accomplished over time and should not be an inherent expectation conferred with one's graduate degree or licensure or experience at a clinic, hospital, or managed care institution. Supervision by a competent and successful individual or group can fill in these missing gaps. Be patient with yourself while you master the art and science of being a talented and effective clinician. It is okay to be frightened about venturing into independent practice. Only time, private practice experience, your own psychotherapy, and good supervision will make you feel more and more comfortable.

As a newcomer to private practice, here are some of our suggestions for your own personal preparation for a successful practice.

1. Begin by reviewing for yourself why you decided to go to graduate school for a degree in the first place. What attracted you to the field? What was your image back then of the kind of work you would be doing after graduation? Has your image changed? Why? Sometimes students become redirected during the course of their studies because of shifts in personal interest and awareness of new and broader aspects to the field. These would be positive reasons for changing that initial desire. These would be changes that occurred from positive growth, learning and personal development. If however you have retreated from what you now think were lofty ideas or impossible dreams, you may need to look into why this change happened. Take note if these changes are due to negative and pessimistic thinking that was encouraged by other pessimistic and negative thinkers.

2. Take note of you own attitude about money. For some rare number of us, money is a comfortable topic. For example, in her workshops on marketing, Laurie Kolt (1998) refers to her natural sense of business, which began early in life while selling lemonade. For most of us, however, money is a difficult, conflictual, and loaded topic. Students and new professionals are typically unaccustomed to getting paid while they are interning in clinics and agencies, so they develop an early pattern of providing free or low-fee psychotherapy. This training is simply a behavioral extension of the mental health worker belief that being in a helping profession is antithetical to being paid. We will discuss this issue further in subsequent chapters, but at this point we note that newer professionals often have a great deal of difficulty setting up a fee-paying situation in which money for psychotherapy is discussed with the client and in which one expects payment.

If this describes you, we suggest that you talk with other more seasoned and successful practitioners and carefully read our chapters on money issues.

3. Join your local, state, and national professional associations. Many organizations have special rates for students and for new graduates. Read their newsletters and attend meetings if you can. Become involved in practice-building issues so that you will be knowledgeable concerning the newest efforts for the development and maintenance of private practice. The more experienced psychotherapists will also be useful role models.

4. Building a practice is an ongoing activity and should be seen as a continuing function of your practice. It is not something that you do for the first 3 months of your professional life or for the first year or first 5 years. Practice building should be seen as an enjoyable and often energizing effort, and, although you may wind up doing pro bono work in exchange for increased visibility, you ultimately will get paid back by referrals to your practice.

5. Improve your professional competency through your own therapy and the expansion of knowledge bases and peer group connections. Realize that using an assortment of practice-building strategies is a strategy itself.

6. Be willing to spend time each day or week or month on your practice-building efforts. You may spend quite a number of hours preparing a talk to give at a local church or temple or at a community program. Additionally, you may need to invest several hours in developing the relationship that leads to such invitations. Remember: the more you invest, the higher your return.

7. Consider the advantages and disadvantages of some managed care affiliations as a "just in case" safety net. Each individual is different

(as in psychotherapy) and no one answer is suitable for all. At one end of the continuum, Norine Johnson,[2] President of APA for the term 2001 to 2002, believes that new psychotherapists benefit from signing onto as many panels as possible. This allows for an immediate full practice and income. At the other end is Karen Shore,[3] the President of the National Coalition of Mental Health Professionals and Consumers who believes that psychotherapists should not sign on to any managed care panels. A more practical recommendation would be that, if one were to work for a managed care panel, it should be with the continued awareness that such experiences may work counter to skills you need as a good practice builder and psychotherapist. Practice building time will be wasted on MCO reports, appeals, and waiting on hold on the telephone. Work at coming to terms with the fact that managed care work often limits your treatment abilities.

8. Try to use your professional contacts from your internship and practicum agency settings. Frequently, senior staff from these agencies can be excellent referral sources for you within the community.

9. If you are employed at a clinic or agency, you may want to begin your private practice slowly. Study the techniques that we will be teaching you in later chapters and gradually begin your efforts to build your practice.

10. Develop your own set of work related strategies (professional niche, psychotherapy techniques, clients served) based on who you are and how you enjoy functioning. Enjoy is an important concept here. Although learning frequently requires stretching to arenas where you have never treaded, look for your sense of enjoyment in your new adventures and your new successes. If you are enjoying the process, you will be much more likely to succeed. Give thought to who you are, how you have succeeded until now and what skills you enjoy both personally and professionally.

My (ER) postdoctoral position became my full-time employment while I built my practice. Because it is not usually possible to open a private practice immediately after graduation, it is best to have employment at a clinic or agency or within a group practice while you develop your own practice. As my practice grew, I reduced my employment to half-time for a few years before venturing into full-time private practice. The postdoctoral position/staff position was at the Los Angeles Suicide Prevention Center, an internationally acclaimed center where I was supervised by outstanding psychologists and psychiatrists who also maintained highly successful private practices. My position grew from undergraduate intern to postdoctoral staff and then to program manager and director of internship training. My years and affiliation at this center afforded me both the excellent training and the mentoring or modeling relationship with outstanding practitioners in mental health. Referrals that began to fill my practice came directly from these affiliations and from my own reputation and the recognition that began to emerge.

I remember making an effort to use all of my earlier training in addition to the most recent because I did not want to be identified solely as an expert on depression and suicide. For 10 years before I returned to graduate school for my doctorate, I was a school psychologist. I had much experience with parenting issues and divorce and separation. I sought to increase my knowledge and exposure to family issues and became a trained stepparenting counselor. Since I also had training in postdivorce court-ordered work I volunteered as a supervisor at a postdivorce family clinic. My intention was to have a general practice for individuals and couples. That is what I still do today.

The time I spent taking additional training in specialty areas and in volunteering to do psychoeducational parenting groups or drug talks at schools in consulting with teachers, or in supervising psychology graduate students was time very well spent developing my name recognition and, bottom line, my practice. I was never paid for any of this work, but I always enjoyed it and was invigorated by it. Did it result in referrals that day or that week? Only sometimes. I do know that it mattered over time. I also feel very certain that had I started in managed care work back then, I never would have had the time to devote to these practice-building efforts that became the foundation of my practice. I would probably not even have gained name recognition as a provider for the clerk at the end of the phone line at the managed care company.

For me (SH), the development of my private practice was combined with other primary employment. My very first patients came from student and colleague referrals when I was a full-time instructor at Brooklyn College, CUNY. When budget cuts came and I was forced to stop teaching, I was offered a position as the Director of Psychological Services at a medical weight loss center. The exposure to this specific group of patients generated a number of referrals, including the patients themselves, their friends, and family members. The referrals were sufficient to give me a solid part-time practice. I really enjoyed working at the weight loss center and became interested in the psychological experience of those patients who had lost a great deal of weight. I decided to gather data on these patients and was able to present the work at an American Psychological Association (APA) meeting. It was my first APA presentation, and it was titled *Fear of Thinness*. To my surprise, this paper was picked up by the United Press International (UPI), and a summary ran in most major newspapers across the country and in *Psychology Today* magazine. Numerous radio and magazine interviews continued through the next few years. The media exposure generated enough patients for me to go into full-time private practice. As I look back, my experience leads me to offer the following advice:

1. Have some consistent form of part-time employment so that you can set about building your direct pay practice without feeling frantic.
2. Choose a specialty area.
3. Try to see enough patients in this niche (even if you have to do it for free) so that you accumulate solid experience.
4. Put your experiences together and generate "talking points" suitable for interesting freebies: media-related articles; synagogue and church workshops; and hospital offerings to the public, college campuses, talks, and so on.
5. If possible, generate a small research study in your chosen area and have it published. This does not need to be in a peer-reviewed journal; rather, it can be in a small newsletter or magazine that is written for professionals involved in your area of specialization. Use copies of this article as handouts when you speak (it increases your credibility), cite it in media articles, and use it in your personal marketing.

My private practice (IL) was an outgrowth of my psychoanalytic training at the Manhattan Institute for Psychoanalysis and my employment in an outpatient psychiatry and developmental center. I began my private practice after many years as a clinical social work supervisor. Although I was not a new clinician, I was very new to starting a private practice. I continued to work full time in my clinic-based position while I built a private practice for about 5 years. It was a slow process, developing a practice, for me even though my work colleagues and community contacts were able to make some referrals. I happily accepted all referrals because I felt that people who knew my work really trusted me. My initial referrals were usually for clients that the referrer did not want.

Neighbors and friends who were in the field of mental health also made referrals. Often, they were individuals who were problematic or who could pay only very low fees. Sometimes they were clients whom others did not have the expertise to see, in other words, handicapped people. My psychoanalytic institute required that I see clients two and three times a week. In order to meet this requirement, I also accepted clients from everywhere I could, including from the Institute's low fee clinic, where I did initial intake interviews without charge. In addition, I worked as consultant field work supervisor for two graduate schools of social work, supervising graduate students who did not have accredited on-site supervision. These students often referred friends and colleagues for either treatment or supervision or both. This led to several private pay supervisees whom I continue to enjoy as a part of my practice.

I was able to develop a full-time practice by becoming involved and networking within organizations, in other words, the New York State Society of Clinical Social Work, American Mental Health Alliance-NY, National Association of Social Workers, and alumni groups. At this time my practice includes work with clients, as a consultant to organizations that need my social work and psychoanalytic skills, and as a connection to a few managed care companies and employee assistance programs. Creating an independent practice has taken a consistent amount of work attending courses, conferences, and seminars and fostering relationships with colleagues.

We hope you have concluded that there are many ways to begin a private practice, and each will be unique to your own set of circumstances. Development of a full-time private practice does take time and is most likely achieved over many months while you are also employed by a school, agency or clinic. As your practice grows, perhaps you can reduce your hours at the agency to half time. Some psychotherapists like to remain on staff at a school or agency because of the sense of security or for the flow of referrals. Mostly, the process of building your independent practice is about finding the opportunities, keeping your eyes open to the possibilities, and accepting the potential that we all have.

We hope that by now you sense our optimism for your ability to succeed in a private pay psychotherapy practice. Nationally, there is a huge wave of students and new graduates in the fields of psychology, social work, and psychiatric nursing. We are certain that there is a population to be served. The following chapters will present you with more alternatives and choices for you to find the most comfortable and enjoyable path to your success as a private practitioner.

NOTES

[1] Personal communication, February 1, 1999.
[2] Personal communication, June 5, 1999.
[3] Personal communication, June 12, 1999.

REFERENCE

Kolt, L. (1998, June 20). How to build a thriving practice today and into the 21st century. Workshop conducted in Los Angeles, CA.

Chapter 3

Fast-Food Psychotherapy

Whether you learned about managed care in graduate school, were presented with it at your clinic or hospital, or were a seasoned therapist recruited by a solicitous letter, at first it probably seemed alright. As unsuspecting professionals, we were unaware of the power that the MCOs would eventually possess and the effect this would have on psychotherapy.

The shocking reality is that managed care has reduced psychotherapy to a tentative connection between professional and patient. The foundation of a working alliance based on privacy, trust, and confidentiality can no longer be guaranteed. In most "talking therapies," the clinical relationship is an essential part of the treatment. This relationship is a dyadic partnership between a client coming to share devastating feelings and chronic uncertainties and a therapist with skill, experience, knowledge, and the ability to understand the intricate and overwhelming issues that are presented. The therapeutic relationship for some becomes reparative, for others a place where intolerable thoughts and wishes can be expressed, and for others a safe haven where interpersonal and intrapsychic concerns are revealed.

Managed care has eroded this therapeutic relationship. Now there is a third person in every consulting room. An MCO case manager is a cost manager whose training may be as a corporate vice president (VP), a business manager, or an administrative assistant. This economic strategy has transformed itself into a mythology about the nature and purpose of clinical work. People who have never seen a client are deciding on the scope of treatment and the number of sessions that are allowed. They are choosing a professional referral based on nothing more that the client's zip code.

The MCO uses a short-term and ultra-brief treatment model. The focus of treatment has shifted to symptom relief, self-help groups, and medication. Patients who do not fit into these classifications are defined as untreatable. Case managers use a number of strategies to monitor the clinician. Their guidelines attempt to contain treatment with "medically necessary" criteria that are further corrupted by fiscal needs. The case manager becomes not just the overseer of costs but also the supervisor of treatment, the judge of the severity of the problems, and the enforcer of standards.

Managed care forces us to face that we are no longer delivering quality care because care is often determined by a clerk, not the patient or the therapist. A typical example is the case of Mary, referred to me by her managed care company. Mary was a 50-year-old depressed, talented, award-winning musician who was unable to translate her musical talent into financial rewards.

For the first 3 months, Mary paid the copayment and I forwarded the remaining bill to the managed care company. For a while, things were fairly straightforward. Then 1 day I received a call instructing me to discuss the case with an insurance company reviewer. It was the beginning of compromises and conflicts in caring.

First, I encountered instructions on the insurance company's answering machine asking me to leave detailed information on their tape; the message assured me that the information was listened to only by the case manager.

When I finally reached the case manager, she told me that the company was tired of paying the bills. They wanted my patient on medication. They wanted her finished with therapy.

I therefore spoke to the patient. She had a strong aversion to medication. She was a politician's wife and was concerned about the stigma of medication.

The relationship with the case manager became antagonistic. My patient and I were losing the battle. I needed evidence of medical necessity to continue our work and I did not have it. Should I make her symptoms sound more serious than they actually were?

Eventually, she accepted a psychiatric consult to appease the managed care company and buy herself more time in therapy. She thought she could schedule the consult a few weeks in advance, take her time filling the prescription, and then not take the medication. Alarmingly, a good portion of our sessions began to be about her wishes to manipulate the insurance company. During these discussions, the patient's husband was unexpectedly relocated and, to our mutual sorrow but the delight (I am sure) of the insurance company, our sessions were brought to an abrupt halt.

Mary's treatment brought up some troublesome issues that question the quality of care:

- Should a therapist and patient collude against a managed care system in order to achieve more treatment for the patient?
- Should a therapist make a patient sound sicker than he or she really is to extend the number of treatment sessions?
- Should a therapist knowingly permit a patient to see a psychiatrist for medication that she or he will not be using?
- Should a patient's wish not to be medicated be honored and defended by the therapist?

These are just some of the ethical problems that arise when the client and the therapist are depersonalized. Central clinical issues of patient autonomy, self-determination, consent, and confidentiality are ignored (see Edward, 1999; Wineburg, 1998).

As psychotherapists participating in managed care programs we are forced to make some serious decisions. How will you treat your patients? Will your treatment decisions be based on your education and training or on the ability to receive payment for your work? To whose contract will you be loyal—your client's or the MCO's? Who decides on the treatment plan? Some MCOs have discharged therapists who have vigorously advocated for their client or who see the necessity of long-term treatment or both. If you want to work with a patient and the patient wants to work with you, how can you do it and still receive adequate compensation? What happens when patients have reached their maximum number of allocated sessions and you have a "duty to do no harm"? Will you be delivering quality care?

Studies indicate that managed care treatment uniformly interferes with the psychotherapy process. Miller (1996) reports one study in which 64% of psychologists reported incidents of MCOs discontinuing treatment when it was still indicated and another study that reported 57% of psychologists saying that their clients' progress had been damaged by managed care denials. A third study found that 90% of the psychologists reported that managed care reviewers interfered with treatment plans that were in the best interests of the client.

Perhaps it should be no surprise that all of the professional disciplines involved with psychotherapy are amassing a body of evidence that clearly supports the efficacy of direct pay psychotherapy as the superior form of treatment. Throughout our lives, we have been taught that "you get what you pay for." Psychotherapy is no exception to this rule. In fact, a study by Hall (1999) on suicidal patients found that many of the would-be suicides would have simply slipped through the cracks if the managed care criteria for hospital admission had been adhered to. In other words, a suicidal patient who does not meet the "official criteria" for hospital admission can be turned away, even when the supervising therapist believes that there are clear indicators of suicidal intent.

The last, and perhaps the most powerful, contribution to the body of objective evidence supporting the quality of direct pay psychotherapy is the landmark study by *Consumer Reports* (Mental Health, 1995) executing the largest mental health survey ever done to assess the everyday consumer's experience and satisfaction with psychotherapy. Four thousand readers were queried about their experiences with mental health care. Their responses formed the data for a mental health report card that clearly grades in favor of long-term therapy outside of the typical managed care packages.

> The longer people stayed in therapy, the more they improved. This suggests that limited mental health insurance coverage, and the new trend in health plans—emphasizing short-term therapy—may be misguided. . . . In our survey of mental health care, respondents whose coverage limited the length and frequency of therapy and the type of therapy, reported poorer outcomes. (*Consumer Reports*, 1995, p. 738)

Our conclusion is that effective and ethical psychotherapy can only happen when there is honesty on the part of the therapist and the patient. It is clear to us that the intrusion of managed care into the treatment process has an adverse effect and undermines the basic tenets of trust that are the sine qua non of psychotherapy. "One size fits all" therapy is not any more effective than is fast food a nutritious diet. Our professional decision is that partnering with managed care no longer seems okay.

> As a parent I know that our goal is to teach our children values. We hope, and pray, that this training will stay with them throughout life. They may modify the values, but we hope that the underlying foundation we have given them remains strong.
>
> Let's now put this in the context of our current situation. As we studied for our doctorates we were trained in a model of psychotherapy. When we graduated many of us went on to postgraduate psychotherapeutic training programs to strengthen our training. No matter whether you are a cognitive behavioral therapist like me or of another orientation we learned certain values. We learned to respect patients. We learned that in the first several weeks of therapy we should identify the problem, build a working rapport, and begin to train the client in what they need to do to benefit from psychotherapy. Psychotherapy is a uniquely personal

experience and takes time. Along comes mangled care. They try to impose a model on us that is totally foreign to the training values that were instilled in us. Their idea of psychotherapy bears little resemblance to what I love to do and was trained to do. The question now is will we sit back and defer to them or strive to regain our professional integrity, and serve patients as we believe is fitting.

Since I am a realist and must support my family, I will only slowly fade out my involvement with mangled care as I replace my income with programs I am developing in a related area—preventive health care. I do have a dream. That dream is to replace my income to the point that I can devote a part of my practice to performing psychotherapy at a very reasonable fee to select patients.

I encourage all who believe in the therapeutic models we were taught to consider alternatives to mangled care.[1]

So, the forces of managed care have left us with several problems that require that we face our issues with money so we can deliver the quality of care that we value and have been trained to deliver. No longer can we delude ourselves into believing that made up fees will keep our caring pure. Our fees are compromised and so is our treatment. The illusion is gone. Ultimately, perhaps, facing these realities will serve us well.

NOTE

[1] D. J. Alne, personal communication, 1999.

REFERENCES

Edward, J. (1999, Spring). Is managed mental health treatment psychotherapy. *Clinical Social Work Journal, 27,* 87–102.

Hall, R. (1999). Suicide risk assessment: A review of risk factors for suicide in 100 patients who made severe suicide attempts. *Psychosomatics, 40,* 18–27.

Miller, I. J. (1996). Managed care is harmful to outpatient mental health services: A call for accountability. *Professional Psychology: Research and Practice, 27*(4), 349–363.

Staff. (1995, November). Mental health: Does therapy help? *Consumer Reports,* pp. 734–739.

Wineburg, M. (1998, Winter). Ethics, managed care and outpatient psychotherapy. *Clinical Social Work Journal, 26,* 433–443.

Part II

All About Money

Chapter 4

Money Matters

In developing a successful private psychotherapy practice, it is critical to recognize that our avoidance and denial of the fact that money matters is the single biggest stumbling block to a successful private-pay practice. All too often, avoidance of money matters is the single biggest stumbling block to the patient's successful psychotherapy experience. For most of us, discussion of money is as taboo today as discussing sex was in Freud's era. In this chapter, we will give voice and challenge beliefs about this all too often ignored issue. We will ask you to reflect on your personal experiences with money, and we will discuss the issue of money as it relates to your professional training and professional experiences.

To begin your internal conversation, we ask you to consider how the following issues have an impact on your behaviors and values.

- Consider the effect of the actual level of your parents' financial success, their satisfaction with that level of success, and their response to the financial milieu on both your conscious and your unconscious attitude towards money. Some families feel that they have enough money; other families feel that there is never enough money. Frequently, these feelings are independent of actual income. As children we often identify with different family members and their roles as provider, healer, nurturer, or savior and incorporate the salient money attitudes attendant to each of these roles.

- Consider that some money anxieties may actually reflect ambivalence. This ambivalence may be about success and accomplishment, particularly when there is an underlying fear or rejection of the autonomy and independence that often go along with success. Unconsciously, there may be the wish that trustworthy others will make your decisions and take care of you, providing longed-for nurturance and caretaking.

• Notice any feelings of unworthiness that a business success can trigger. In particular, we note that financial success can stimulate underlying conflict about competition and an uncomfortable sense of doing better than one's parents, sibling, and colleagues.

• Creating wealth for oneself may conflict with an ethical upbringing that stresses values of altruism, humane sacrifice, and selflessness. Even if you do not identify with such an upbringing, you probably decided to go into the field of mental health to "help people."

Now, consider your professional training. Reflect on your graduate school experiences. Your years in graduate school probably helped you to avoid money anxieties by continuing the one-dimensional caring myth. You probably had no courses on marketing, although there were no doubt plenty of classes on the "individual and society," "personality development," and "cross-cultural differences." Did anybody in any of these classes ever mention that eventually you would have to earn a living? Did anyone ever say that "helping people" is a wonderful life value but carries no weight with a mortgage company? Did anyone, anywhere, ever talk to you about the basics of operating a business?

Finally, honestly reflect on your professional experiences. When was the last time you went to a professional conference and any of the speakers discussed money? Have you ever attended a symposium on countertransference and heard therapists talk about envying their patients' income and lifestyle? How often has a colleague confided in you what his or her bottom line income was for the year?

Our guess is that none of this has happened to you very often. Perhaps, it has never happened at all. Strange is it not? Did you ever notice that this strange cultlike silence exists for most everyone in the mental health profession when it comes to the topic of money? We have adopted the mind-set that money taints our altruism, sullies our purity, and makes our motives suspect. Life realities of rent, food, and personal desires live somewhere other than in the therapy room. Secretly, however, many of us covet our colleagues' higher fees, envy our patients' wealth and freedom, and resent a life of doing without.

Within our profession, the emphasis is on empathy and understanding. We learned to value caring and nurturing. We identify with the disadvantaged and the less privileged. Focusing on money can feel like a threat to our career choice. We fear that we will be seen as uncaring and unconcerned. We choose to help our patients by throwing a personal lifeline offering our support, skills, and empathy. In our efforts to strengthen our patients, however, we do not ask for their money. Rather, we view our fees as a drain on their very limited resources. We choose not to participate in this hurtful process. How in good conscience can we take from others and call it caring? In many ways we feel like an impostor. We are charging for a service that should be free. Many of us are caught up in the conundrum of financial ambivalence.

There is no easy resolution to the money–caring dilemma, although at some point every caring person faces the fact that sometimes caring is the act of "not giving." There is a proverb about teaching a man to fish rather than giving him a fish. The former is a skill that lasts a lifetime; the latter, a momentary fix. There is also no question in the moment that it would be easier to simply give the man a fish. "Easy" is not always the answer. Giving away therapy does not teach people how to feed and fend for themselves. Money—the ability to earn it, ask for it, and expect it—is deeply related to the experience of self-esteem. How much is my service really worth? How much am I really worth? How can we build a patient's self-esteem with a service that is not intrinsically worthy? How can we build a patient's self-esteem when the therapist does not feel that he or she is intrinsically worthy?

> Once I had this dream. I remember that I had an image of myself standing in Manhattan by the East River. I had achieved some fame and this picture of me by the river was on the *New York Times Magazine* cover. But, I looked down and saw myself in my old fuddy-duddy social work shoes. My analyst suggested that it was about my conflict and ambivalence between being the woman of the year or one of the neediest cases. It was a conflict between giving and taking.[1]

Then there are our personal worries. We are worried about how the patient will feel about us. We are concerned about being liked and are afraid of being rejected or being perceived as not kind enough.

The truth is that it is healthy and appropriate to want to make money. To a large degree we determine our income by setting our fees. The forces that inhibit our success are internal and are related to personal issues of authority, acceptance, ownership, and fear of rejection. We need to determine the expenses of our private practice and the value of our services. We are working for ourselves, and establishing a fee is a practical matter. Our comfort, honesty, and openness about money can serve as a frame for our own and the client's personal exploration and development concerning money. A therapist with conflicts about money may have a blind spot for the same issue in the patient or may resent a patient's desire for success, achievement, and money.

The independent practice of psychotherapy offers a unique opportunity for professional financial success. We leave you with Freud's helpful reminder: He notes that the treatment would not work without a fee. Since the analyst had an effective method, an expensive fee was appropriate (Freud, 1949).

300.xx DSM IV vs. PROFIT ANXIETY

Diagnostic Feature

The essential feature of a profit anxiety disorder is the presence of marked anxiety and guilt in collecting profitable fees for the delivery of psychological services. This disorder, prevalent amongst psychologists, usually manifests itself in adulthood, some time after the completion of graduate school.

Subtypes

Profit anxiety may be present but asymptomatic for psychologists working in institutions or other salaried positions (i.e., academia, clinics, hospitals).

In these cases, the disorder can be ascertained by the prevalence of anger or envy of colleagues who have part-time psychotherapy practices. Symptoms will be fully manifest if the individual opens a private practice, at which time there may be overt or masked envy at patients who dress well and take frequent vacations.

Associated Features and Disorders

There may be discontent with occupational functioning, preoccupation with money issues, and the presence of both masochistic and altruistic tendencies.

Specific Culture, Age and Gender Features

This disorder appears widespread and is not restricted to any one cohort.

Prevalence

There is widespread prevalence among all psychologists, with manifest symptoms more pronounced among independent practitioners.

Differential Diagnosis

Not to be confused with depression.

One could say with some certainty that to be a psychotherapist is to be ambivalent and anxious about money.

Most therapists originally entered the profession with a calling to help humanity. We share some blend of ethics, altruism, caring and a wish to use these skills to improve society. Somewhere along the way, this wish was deemed to be incompatible with financial profit. For many years, this conflict remained asymptomatic. The condition was managed through third party payments. Therapists usually only had to collect modest copayments, and patients usually did not have a significant financial responsibility for their psychological treatment. Today, this arrangement has changed, and the successful psychotherapist in private practice has a direct fee paying relationship with their patients. To be successful, financial ambivalence needs to be resolved. Here is one contribution to this resolution.

Most psychotherapists do not link the success and wealth of their business with the time, energy, and resources they have to reinvest in the world at large. In a linkage model, career success ensures a mechanism to improve society. Without career success, work and financial anxiety consume the waking hours, stultify creative energy, and limit altruistic gifts.

So, with the values of caring and social change as the foundation, I ask you to begin to think about money so that your competence can improve the lives of as many people as possible. With a positive attitude towards profit, we can construct a win-win-win situation. The mental health professional acquires money, lives a comfortable life, and feels successful about work. The patient is the recipient of focused attention, thoughtful, personalized interventions, and a dose of unpressured, unhurried expertise. Society reaps the benefits of your increased energy, time, and financial resources. (Haber, 1998, pp. 62–63)

NOTE

[1] J. Bristol, personal communication, December 11, 1999.

REFERENCES

Freud, S. (1949). Further recommendations on technique. In *Collected papers,* vol. 2; J. Strachey, Ed. & Trans.). London: Hogarth Press. (Original work published 1913)

Haber, S. (1998). Profit anxiety. *Independent Practitioner, 18*(2), 62–63.

Chapter 5

How to Ask for Money and How to Get It

B y now, you may be concluding that underneath it all you have a few unresolved money issues. Perhaps you are also convinced that managed care's version of caring has nothing to do with caring. Hopefully, you are determined to conquer your conflicts so you can earn good money and deliver the quality care your patients deserve.

Changing your relationship with money and transferring this change to your patients often involves psychodynamic processes. We addressed these processes in chapter 4 by asking you to reflect on your motives. Now that your personal motives are clarified, the subsequent steps necessary to actualize your money-making behaviors will be facilitated by cognitive and behavioral changes. In this chapter, we offer a number of suggestions you can use to develop and expand your direct pay psychotherapy practice.

PEOPLE CAN PAY FOR PSYCHOTHERAPY

The fundamental starting point for your private-pay psyche needs to be the unshakable belief that many people can afford to pay for psychotherapy services. This country has a vast middle-class and upper-middle-class population that has access to discretionary income. Now this does not mean that they want to spend their money on psychotherapy; it merely means that they are able to do so—if and when they choose. To get a feeling for the amount of money people will spend on promising health-related services, consider the booming field of alternative medicine. Recent data tell us that one out of three people each year is perfectly willing to spend out of pocket dollars for nonreimbursed health care to treat a serious or bothersome problem— to the tune of more than 10 billion dollars. Clearly, many people are able to pay for health-related services and products.

In solidifying your beliefs about your patients' ability to pay, remember to review how your patients spend money. Reflect on their big ticket purchases, such as vacations, children's camps, plastic surgery, landscaping, car purchases, and home improvements. Be sure to consider the smaller, repetitive, mindless, routine expenses—the "Cash Without Question" expenses—including manicures, beauty salons, dry cleaners, gym memberships, yoga classes, movie theaters, ice cream stores, and restaurants. These services are routinely used by the same patients who do not want to pay your full fee.

Tennis lessons $90 per hour
Homework tutor $75 per hour
Speech therapist $80 per hour
Personal trainer $60 per hour
Hairdressers $35–135 depending upon the service
Psychic reading $70 per hour

Another helpful mind management technique for strengthening your money resolve is to remind yourself why people seek your services. Often, there is a presenting problem that is far more expensive than your treatment. For example, if a patient is seeing you for a smoking problem, remember that a carton of cigarettes is about $30 to $35. A two pack a day smoker's habit costs more than $50 per week, close to the cost of psychotherapy at the low end of a sliding scale. Therapy to quit smoking is more short term and will end up saving the person thousands and thousands of dollars as well as years of illness, medical expenses, and an earlier death. Full fee charges for this type of patient is a cost-effective investment for the patient and the patient's family.

Food addicts have even pricier habits. Depending on the level of overeating (junk versus gourmet food), the costs of overeating can be minimally estimated as an extra $20 per day. This easily adds up to at least $140 per week, a respectable psychotherapy fee in most areas of the country. Periodic attempts by food addicts to diet are also very costly; diet centers and diet programs are typically not covered by insurance.

Shopping is another very expensive habit. In addition to rushing to the mall after a bad day, or a good day, shopping addicts now also have easy access to spending their dollars via shopping through the television and Internet. There is no question that full fee psychotherapy can save these patients thousands of dollars in the long run.

Last, cocaine is perhaps the most expensive addiction. Cocaine addicts spend thousands of dollars, lose their homes, and steal from their relatives to support their habits. They will and should pay for full fee therapy when they are truly motivated to kick their habit. There should be no question that they can "afford" your services.

PSYCHOTHERAPY IS COST-EFFECTIVE

In addition to addictions, there are many other areas in which psychotherapy is cost-effective. Marital therapy is an example. A couple's serious commitment to psychotherapy can save a crumbling marriage. Although the therapy bill may seem high, the cost is mere pennies when compared with attorney and dissolution costs, court fees, and years of postdivorce anguish. It is helpful to remember that attorney fees are universally higher per hour than are psychotherapy fees; cost effectiveness is no contest.

Patients with psychosomatic symptoms who do not enter the psychotherapy office frequently wind up filling medical waiting rooms. Their illnesses create physician costs, prescription costs, losses in individual earnings, and losses in company profits. These cumulative costs are far more expensive than is the cost of psychotherapy.

In the business arena, executives with character problems both limit a company's productivity and create interpersonal conflicts that can result in costly employee turnover. "Executive coaching" or psychotherapy with such individuals is a cost-effective way of managing these issues. Promising employees with self-defeating psychological issues often never achieve their potential. Paying to address these issues has a positive return on investment in the long run.

In the previous examples, both psychotherapists and patients are accustomed to spending thousands of dollars on drugs, attorney fees, medical tests, and lost income. It is important for you, the independent psychotherapist, to be clear that your service, although perceived as expensive, is unquestionably cost-effective for your clients.

Once you are solid in your fundamental beliefs that many people can pay for psychotherapy services and that such services are cost-effective, you should address the issue of the quality of care you can deliver. Simply put, you can deliver a better quality psychotherapy service if you are directly paid by your patient.

PRIVATE PAY BUYS CONFIDENTIALITY

When a patient pays for psychological services it protects the fundamental principle that underlies all good treatment; confidentiality. Other
than in the mandated instances of suicide, homicide, and child abuse,
the personal issues revealed to the therapist paid directly are protect-
ed by law.

After confidentiality is corrupted (as in the managed care situation),
the patient is less likely to disclose information that is embarrassing or
shameful. There will be much conscious editing of what is brought to
the therapy session. We can assume that without confidentiality there
will be little access to the unconscious processes that are uncovered
during the course of psychotherapy.

Kremer and Gesten (1998) explored varying levels of therapeutic
confidentiality and related these levels to willingness to disclose. Findings
indicated significantly less willingness to disclose in a managed care
setting as compared with a standard fee for service condition. "The
ineffectiveness of the persuasive rationale suggests that it will be very
difficult for psychologists to overcome their managed care clients'
concerns about the loss of confidentiality in therapy" (pp. 555–556).

YOUR ANXIETY ABOUT GETTING PAID

So now you, the directly paid therapist, know that many people can pay
for your services and that these services are cost-effective. You also
believe that in your direct pay practice you will be delivering a higher
quality service that protects the confidentiality of the patient. Now, we
move on to discuss the need for anxiety reduction. Although each of us
has unique concerns about developing a private-pay practice; a nearly
universal anxiety is the financial uncertainty of private practice without
(or limiting) the safety net of a managed care company. It is important
to reduce this anxiety so that you have the freedom to turn away
patients; raise your fees; resign from one, several, or all managed care
panels or simply have time to develop and implement creative marketing endeavors. Your anxiety can best be controlled by reducing expenses and maximizing income. Here are some options to consider:

- Reduce expenses by considering a home office, a shared office,
  or a sublet office. One creative therapist we know in a major city
  sublets her office on weekends as a bed and breakfast. After carefully locking away her files, she provides a convertible couch,
  linens, and coffee maker.

- Replace the managed care referral safety net with steady part time income such as from adjunct teaching. Remember that part-time jobs also serve to increase your visibility in the community and will help you generate referrals.
- Choose to maintain an affiliation with a few of the less intrusive preferred provider organizations but save your prime hours for direct pay patients.
- Consider offering a nonreimbursed service to both your managed care and your direct pay patients. For example, an educational workshop in changing careers, parenting your adolescent children, or building self-esteem are not services covered by managed care companies. You are usually free to generate additional monies from managed care clients, as long as they are not from psychotherapy services.
- Join a mental health cooperative of professionals or a guild. These organizations affiliate multiple disciplines in a joint effort to arrange for the delivery of mental health services by their members (examples include American Mental Health Alliance [AMHA]-USA; Connecticut Guild, Boulder Guild). Recently, it was reported in the *Wall Street Journal* that

> The Connecticut Psychotherapist's Guild now offers a safe haven from managed care, which has slashed therapist's fees, curtailed patient treatment and, for many, turned mental health into one of the gloomiest realms in US health care. . . . Those who have joined a guild or one of the similar loose-knit organizations that have sprung up in at least 10 regions around the county subscribe to a simple tenet: patients are fed up with the current system and will pay for treatment out-of-pocket as long as rates are reasonable. (Murray, 1999)

- Become active in your local professional organizations and help organize a network. On a local level you can participate in the creation of a referral network among members. The more involved you are, the more likely you are to become know as a professional in the community.
- Get involved in your institute or university mental health clinical referral services. By offering to work for low fees, doing administrative work, and conducting intakes for no or low fees, you will be able to build your practice and fill hours. By participating in the clinic, you may also be privy to low fee supervision.

By taking some of the actions just listed, you will be able to reduce your anxiety and free up needed energy and creativity for use in your direct pay practice.

Finally, you will also need to diminish your guilt. We recognize that the deep-seated conflict between caring and money does not simply disappear. So, if guilt management is necessary consider the following suggestion. Keep business and charity separate. Focus on the fact that the more you earn, the fewer patients you need to see. With more time available, make a commitment to give away your caring through pro bono work (perhaps at a different location or only during specific hours) or through volunteer activities separate from your direct fee practice.

Consider the following "guilt management scenario" (Haber, 1998).

> Let's assume you need to earn $1000. At a typical managed care rate, this requires 14 patient hours at $75 per session. At a typical fee-for-service rate it requires 10 patient hours at $100 per session. At a niche specialty that is doing well, you only need 7 patient hours at $150 per session. For the super expert with great skills and great marketing, the workload is only 5 patient hours at $200 per session.
>
> Translated into a day with the typical break for lunch, this means that the managed care therapist works from 8 AM until 11 PM, the average therapist works from 8 AM until 7 PM, the niche specialist works from 8 AM until 4 PM, and the super skills/super marketer works from 8 AM until a 1 PM lunch.
>
> In the managed care situation you would not have much time for caring, skill building, creative thinking, or anything else, including your family. You will have been charitable to those 14 patients, many of whom may not have needed your charity. In the average case, you have worked a full day and can have dinner with your family. Both the specialist and the super expert can work a half day, provide pro bono service in their community, keep up with the literature, and have dinner with the family. I suggest that it is the latter two groups of practitioners who, in the long run, contribute more to society.

HOW TO ASK FOR PAYMENT

With a strong foundation of private pay beliefs, reduced anxiety and guilt, and a support system of confident colleagues, you can "practice your lines." Here are several ways to deal with money questions that come up in practice:

- State your fee by saying; "My usual fee is $X per hour." If you are on the phone and hear a pause or if you are speaking in person and you see a disappointed look, say; "This is my full fee. If this is not possible for you I do have a sliding scale." (You can refer the client to a colleague at this point if you choose not to have a sliding scale.) You can also ask, "What fee did you have in mind when you decided to come to therapy?" If the patient responds with a fee at the very low end of your acceptable range, you can counteroffer with "is it possible for you to pay $X?" Usually this is close enough to the client's budget that he or she can stretch to this; if not, you can accept the suggested fee. You can close the discussion by saying that you prefer keeping the arrangement flexible. If the client should have difficulty maintaining this fee, it will need to be discussed. If the client receives a large increase in income, it is expected that the fee will be increased. This is usually seen as a mutually fair negotiation, and the first appointment can be set. If the patient cannot afford your sliding fee, then you need to refer him or her to a colleague.

• If a patient is having financial problems, participating in a psychotherapy group can be cost-effective and therapeutic. Consider having at least one group in your practice to provide an additional treatment modality as well as easing financial constraints. Generally, a well-run group can be immensely helpful to patients and can be offered at a fee that is substantially lower than that for individual treatment. Individuals can attend group along with individual sessions on a regular, semi-regular, or as-needed basis.

• If questioned about a high fee, you can say the following: "Yes, you are paying a high fee. You have one of the higher incomes in my practice so you, and several others, are paying the most. People who earn less pay less. If the day comes when you lose your job and cannot pay a high fee, I will be able to offer you a similar reduction until you are back on your feet."

• If you are taking a managed care patient, you might want to tell him or her what your usual fee is in the first session: "As part of plan x, you will be allowed a number of sessions and will only be responsible for a small co-pay. However, you do need to know that if you want additional sessions after the allotted number, my fee is X."

• If you are asked in an initial phone call whether you are on a managed care plan, you need to be straightforward. You can add a brief commercial, in other words, "I am not on MC panel X. If you find the treatment offered from your policy to be too limited, feel free to call me back." If you know why the patient is seeking treatment and happen to offer specialized services you can say, "I am not on MC panel X, but you are probably covered for a few sessions. You might want to know that I offer a half-day workshop in topic X. You can call me if you are interested, or, if you would like, I will send you some information now."

• The issue of raising fees is frequently avoided by even the most experienced therapists. Once over the anxiety of fee negotiation and fee setting, there is a huge sigh of relief, and most feel glad not to have to return to this issue. There are many who never raise their fee and charge the same fee for many years. Interestingly, some feel that it is okay to raise the fee for new patients but have difficulty raising the fees of ongoing patients.

If you have difficulty with the issue of fee increases consider an annual increase of $5.00 per year for all patients. Generally speaking, there will be little resistance to this. Those paying a high full fee have no difficulty in making this change, and the patients paying lower fees usually feel very comfortable and glad to be able to pay a bit more. Of course, if there are special circumstances, there is the flexibility for discussion and negotiation.

For the student or young professional just beginning in private-pay practice, the previous conversations may feel very scary. You may feel that you have no right in asking for a fee above what you were accustomed to having at the local mental health clinic where you interned. Unfortunately, most clinics and training venues do not include fee setting as part of their training. An unusual internship training experience is described in the following. As you read it, try to imagine yourself in the same situation and how this training could help you to get the nerve to ask for money.

> During my (ER) internship training I learned that it was important for patients to pay for their therapy, not for the classic psychotherapeutic reasons but as a matter of economic survival for the clinic. The clinic in which I worked provided court-ordered psychotherapy for divorced couples who were resistant to judicial decisions regarding spousal support or child custody. Some of these couples had been divorced for years yet were continuing their battles and refusing to cooperate to fulfill their legal commitments. Clearly these were difficult patients. The clients hated each other, hated being told that they had to attend psychotherapy, and hated that they needed to pay for it. Frequently, sessions were ended abruptly by one exspouse walking out in a huff. Because the requirement was that each spouse should pay his or her own portion, the clinic was aware that they might never see that fee. The rule of the clinic was, therefore, that the therapist was to obtain the fee before the session. No payment . . . no session. "Checkbook is in the car." "I'll wait while you go get

it." "I forgot the check." "We'll reschedule the appointment." This was excruciatingly difficult for the interns. The director was adamant, and we felt we would be fired from our internship if we did not follow his orders. So, we learned how to do this quickly. Over time, it became easier and easier, and we learned how important this was to the survival of the clinic. I learned to be comfortable about asking for payment. It taught me to feel entitled to be paid and to be paid an adequate fee.

As a result, my patients pay in a timely manner, and I almost never have accounts that go unpaid.

We suggest that you reread the preceding narrative a few times and use it as a learning experience.

THE STORY OF THE ORGANIC CARROT

Several years ago, I was walking down the main street of my neighborhood. I noted that the health food store was expanding for the third time in the past decade. I entered the store and noted that carrots cost 99¢ a pound. I then left the store and on the very next block came to the neighborhood supermarket, where I found carrots that cost 39¢ a pound.

Both the health food store and the supermarket were doing well—each had its devoted customers—yet the health food store was selling foods for almost three times as much. When one considers a basketful of produce, this becomes a significant difference in expenditure. I wondered, "what makes people willing to pay more for 'seemingly' similar products?"

The answer of course is that the health food store sells organic fruits and vegetables whereas the supermarket sells ordinary (pesticide-sprayed) products. Both items look the same. For many people, both items taste the same. The customers in the health food store believe that the organic foods are healthier, and therefore it is appropriate that they cost three times as much. It is an extension of the belief that you pay for what you get.

Customers who buy organic foods believe they are getting a better product. The organic vegetables may indeed be superior, but, in fact, the evidence is mostly that of face value. But it does not matter because organic products

satisfy the consumers' wish to be healthy. The organic produce has successfully differentiated itself from supermarket
quality produce.

We can learn from this that there are consumers for each
type of product. For some, the price is the key variable. For
others, it is the quality of the product that determines the
purchase. In the latter group, we learn that people will pay
for higher-priced products and services as long as they can
differentiate the higher-priced item as being of superior value.

The same principles underlie marketing independent psychological services. The problem does not rest solely with
the consumer's ability to pay. A good part of the problem
rests in our failure to differentiate ourselves and our product
as superior and worth paying for. Have we made it clear to
the public that independently practicing psychologists are
able to address issues that are untouched by traditional
health care? Have we made it clear that independently practicing psychologists deliver their services while maintaining
patient confidentiality? Have we made it clear that independently practicing psychologists are free to determine and
deliver the optimum course of treatment unhampered by
conflicts of interest from unseen third parties?

The conclusion is obvious. Let us all resolve that from
now on we will address these problems and differentiate our
product to a substantial portion of the public that stands
ready, willing, and able to pay for psychological services.

Think organic carrots! (Haber, 1998, pp. 6–7)

REFERENCES

Haber, S. (1998). Lessons from the organic carrot. *Independent Practitioner,*
18(1), 6–7

Kremer, T. G., & Gesten, E. L. (1998). Confidentiality limits of managed care
and clients' willingness to self-disclose. *Professional Psychology: Research
and Practice, 29*(6), 553–558.

Murray, S. (1999, November 22). Guild therapies choose to abandon managed care. *The Wall Street Journal,* p. B1.

Part III

Carving Your Niche and Marketing Your Services

Chapter 6

Watch Your Language!

What's in a name? What you call yourself and how you describe your services delivers your message. Your message defines you and associates you with a particular situation.

Most people connect the term "psychotherapist" with psychiatrists, psychologists, or counselors. They identify psychotherapists as professionals who work with people who have mental health problems. For those people who readily acknowledge having a mental health problem, seeking the services of a psychotherapist is therefore the logical course of action. However, for many new potential clients, either this is a very uncomfortable way to think, or they are just unaware of the connection between psychotherapy and help with a specific life problem. If, for example, people want to improve an aspect of their life, such as a career change, or seek to master anxiety about meeting new people, they may recognize their need to talk this through with a professional, but they do not feel like they have a "mental problem."

For such individuals, psychotherapy and psychotherapist are an unappealing way to describe your services.

WHO ARE YOU? WHAT DO YOU DO?

Think about the conversation you usually have when a new patient calls to make an appointment. Does the caller begin by asking for psychotherapy for his or her mental problem, or does the conversation go more like this: Caller: "I'm calling because I finally realized that I need help dealing with my anger. Do you work with this problem?" You, if you are cognitive/behavioral: "Yes, I do. I have experience with people who need to learn to control their anger. I can teach you anger management." You, if you are psychodynamic: "Yes, I do help people who feel very angry. I can help you to identify the source of your anger and then help you to work it out so that you are not unknowingly affected by it."

You may find that you are already practicing these kinds of communication skills as you function in your practice, especially when they are framed for you by the prospective patient. We now ask that you own this style yourself and realize that it is a very effective way to communicate who you are and what you do to the public, your prospective clients.

When you first studied for your degree, you probably appreciated the enormous breadth of the mental health field. Psychologists were statisticians, assessors, researchers, and experimenters. Social workers focused on case management, the family and community, linkages and networking, and community resources. A psychotherapist worked with children, adults, groups, and industries. As your training advanced, so did the specifics and intricacies of your professional language.

We learned to be fluent in a layer of language that included processes, objects, cathexis, reframing, and reinforcement to name just a few words and concepts that reflected the particular culture of our respective training institutions. This professional language provided a common basis for our internal collegial dialogues and professional writings. Unfortunately, the professional dialect continues to be used in the outside world where it is significantly less useful, if understood at all.

Most of us are savvy enough to be language conscious during public speaking, although this tends to be through the process of avoidance of jargon rather than through the use of clearer, more operational terms. Even the accepted language of "psychotherapy," "personality change," "ambivalence," "limited affect," or even the euphemistic "getting in touch with" are to most of the public vague descriptions that can seem to be unrelated to the listener's or reader's perceived problem. Such language requires the prospective patient to make a leap between the description you deliver and the problem they would like addressed. For many people this leap is simply too big. So what is a successful, competent private practitioner to do? (Haber, 1998, p. 118)

USING USER-FRIENDLY WORDS

Today you need to recapture the breadth of our original disciplines and return to a simpler language identifiable to that public you would like to serve. In other words, to develop a direct pay psychotherapy practice, you will need to consider repackaging and renaming both the problems you are addressing and the services you are providing to make your practice more user friendly while still maintaining your professionalism. It is much easier to market services that address readily identifiable problems that prospective clients already know they have. These are the clients who are most willing to come to you for help.

What follows are a few examples of specific problems with a few million potential patients just waiting for your services. There are some suggested areas in which you can introduce yourself and talk about what you do in words that listeners can understand and convey to the listeners that you understand them too. There are topics framed in such a manner that your prospective patients can make the leap from their problem, to how *you* can help.

- You may have noticed a high percentage of failed marriages in this country, and many of those that survive exist in a stalemate of misery. Here is a large category of people who need and want marital consulting services. It is quite common for one person in the couple to "want therapy" but the other refuses therapy. A less threatening "service" might be acceptable to that intimidated spouse. A service described as "Marital Communication Skill Building" could open the door to your office.
- Look to children who have learning disabilities or handicaps in schools that are understaffed and overcrowded. Teachers, one of the most underpaid and unacknowledged professionals, simply do not have the time to work with each of these children. Parents are clamoring for a professional who can help their child without further stigma falling on their child.
- Check out the 50 million tobacco addicts in the United States. Tobacco remains the leading preventable cause of death and results in $50 billion of direct medical costs. Unfortunately, the rate of smoking among high school students has increased in recent years to 35% of the high school population. You can team up with a local health club or lung association and offer support and information. Within the corporate world, businesses may be happy to pay for counselors to help their employees stop smoking. However, in these organizations or corporations, presenting yourself as a psychotherapist will not even get

you a conversation on the phone. You will need to frame your service in a manner that is positive and growth promoting. Although you will be offering techniques based on your education and training as a psychotherapist, you will be communicating your specific problem-solving skills that help people quit an unhealthy habit.

• There are 34 million overweight people in the United States. Despite what pharmaceutical houses would like us to believe, obesity that comes from overeating and underexercising is usually due to psychological issues. Check out the cover of almost every major women's magazine to see just how prevalent this concern is to their millions of readers. Yet, how often do you see the recommendation for psychotherapy? Never. Rather, the accepted recommendation is to get vague and unspecified "professional help."

• Much of the population is aging. Groups, seminars, and workshops on the future of the baby boomers have become big business. Psychotherapists have a major role to play in this new emerging arena. Issues can include topics such as retirement, midlife career changes, remarriage, and grandparenting. Consider approaching an adult community or retirement center to offer a series of talks on any of these topics. This population would welcome your services when they are presented in a manner that does not identify aging with illness.

Think about your specialty areas, and the areas in which you enjoy working. Below are some examples of topics that can be tailored to several different populations. Consider these examples, and especially notice the language used in identifying the help that a person can get from a psychotherapist without using the word psychotherapy.

• Helping parents talk to their children (youngsters, preteens, teenager, etc.)
• Teaching patients to communicate with physicians (applicable to populations with different illnesses and in a variety of medical settings)
• Anxiety reduction (for specific situations such as preparation for surgery, to combat fear of flying, or in general stress management)
• Improving motivation to exercise (applicable to overweight individuals, "wellness" communities, and physical rehabilitation)
• Overcoming insomnia
• Managing the difficult toddler or teenager
• Reducing homework horrors (generally suitable for children in the middle years)
• Imagery for success in sports (such as golf or tennis)

- Increasing self-confidence (wide applicability)
- Enhancing work relationships (oriented toward management, getting along with the boss, and collegial relationships)

WHAT TO CALL YOURSELF

In addition to identifying a focal problem and the language you use to describe your service, we also suggest that you consider professional descriptions in addition to that of psychotherapist. All of the preceding were specific problems in which you could deliver your services not only as a psychotherapist but also as a consultant, coach, mentor, adviser, or counselor. One of the most popular and marketable professional services is "coaching." Although coaching and psychotherapy can often be similar services, people will pay big dollars for coaching when they will not reach into their pockets to pay for psychotherapy. The language you use can affect the fee you get. Let us analyze the reasons for this:

- One distinction between psychotherapists and coaches lies in the definitions of the problems they are addressing and the persons they are treating. As we have said, psychotherapy tends to identify problems and flaws within the individual's personality. Coaching, however, is a positive term that is filled with optimism and possibilities.
- Coaching tends to focus on a specific problem with no implied evaluation about the person who has this problem.
- Coaching implies learning over a specific period of time. Psychotherapy tends to be open ended and can often seem to be a process that never comes to a conclusion.
- Coaching implies the promise of a specific outcome. Psychotherapy is usually described in vague terms without such a promise.

A number of mental health professionals have successfully incorporated aspects of coaching into their psychotherapy practices. For example, Arthur Kovacs[1] calls himself a "life transition counselor," a term that describes a mix of psychotherapy and coaching. In his work, Kovacs focuses on life transitions as the points of need for people, offering his services to individuals at all different stages of life. As a life transition counselor, Kovacs remains outside the medical model/managed care system, and his patients avoid the stigma associated with mental illness. Sue Erickson Bloland and Judith Bristol[2] package their services similarly. They began "Mid-Life Mentors," where they offer workshops and seminars on a variety of topics that appeal to clients in the middle years of life.

Richard Trachtman (psychotherapist) and Jan Hopkins Trachtman[3] (financial journalist) used their joint talents to form a service that addresses money and relationships issues. In their respective professions, they realized repeatedly how money affects the way people think, feel, and behave, as well as how the way they think and feel affects how they behave around money. These observations led them to develop MORE Services (an acronym for MOney and RElationships). The word more itself reflects a positive growth process in which the patient or client will have gains.

It should be easy to see why these specific services may have a broader appeal than "psychotherapy" has to many members of the public. Hopefully, it is also clear that once an individual accepts your services for a specific problem, there is a good chance that he or she will become interested in more complex issues. For those of you who are interested in providing long-term psychodynamic treatment, it may be helpful to realize that if you begin with a specific approach you will often be able to gradually educate and interest the patient in the offerings of a more complex, longer-term therapy process. This of course is usually the result of the patient being pleased with the gains he or she is making from the service you were initially providing.

Psychotherapy is probably the backbone of your practice, but most patients do not enter through the psychotherapy door. Rather, the perceived value of psychotherapy seems to require a long educational process that gradually emerges as your relationship with your patients builds. Psychotherapy is your agenda, not necessarily theirs. Psychotherapy can, and frequently does, become the mutual treatment of choice but typically only after the patient's presenting problem has been managed or contained. In other words, you need to address the patient's agenda first.

The most important message to take with you here is that although most people can accept problems in their life, they usually have a much more difficult time accepting that their own personality or self is flawed. Most can accept help from tutors and teachers, counselors and consultants; they have a much more difficult time going to psychotherapists. Most people had a coach in high school or college or knew a coach, or they see coaches on television all the time. Most have not worked with a psychotherapist, and most have not even met a psychotherapist. Remember that the language you use in describing yourself and the work you do causes your office door to open or close.

NOTES

[1] Personal communication, April 13, 1999.
[2] Personal communication, December 11, 1999.
[3] Personal communication, December 10, 1999.

REFERENCES

Erickson Bloland, S., & Bristol, J. (1999). *Mid-life mentors* [Brochure]. Available from J. Bristol (see Appendix).
Haber, S. (1998, Summer). Presidential column. *Independent Practitioner,* pp. 118–119.
Trachtman, R. (1999). *MORE Services for MOney & RElationships* [Brochure]. Available from R. Trachtman (see Appendix).

Chapter 7

Are You a Generalist, Specialist, or Both?

Psychotherapy training begins with a general population of clients. We practiced our craft on adults, children and teens, and older adults. Upon completion of our graduate training and internships we anticipated doing some type of generic therapy or treatment. Most of us began our professional careers in clinics, inpatient units, medical centers, departments of psychiatry, or in community agencies or programs addressing psychological problems in their many different forms.

Through all of our learning and initial work history we became skilled in "general" psychotherapy. Most of us began our private practice with the same idea—that we would see clients from the general population. Our hope was that colleagues would send referrals because they knew us and knew that we did good work. This is a logical way to begin but it is ineffective and unreliable in today's health care economy. To be a successful generalist psychotherapist it is usually easier to begin with a niche, a specialization in which you can distinguish yourself. If you reflect on your more successful colleagues, you will observe that almost all of them have a specialization of one kind or another. Examples of specializations include treatment of non–English speaking clients or clients for whom English is a second language; counseling gay couples; divorce mediation; pain management; and treatment of handicapped clients, to name just a few of the many possibilities.

HOW SPECIALIZATION HELPS DEVELOP A GENERAL PSYCHOTHERAPY PRACTICE

Although some practitioners focus exclusively on their specialty, we also found a number of therapists who only had 10 to 20% of their patients within their specialty area. The specialty simply enables the practitioner to become known in the community and to be suggested as a specific referral source distinct from the other potential referral possibilities for a specific subset of clients.

Often when therapists are considering specialization they become concerned about dilution of their general psychotherapy referrals. For example, they are afraid that if they are identified as a specialist in singles issues patients with anxiety reactions will not seek their services. They may worry that if they are identified as an attention deficit hyperactivity disorder (ADHD) specialist, patients with marital problems will not consider them an appropriate choice. Generally speaking, this does not happen. If you deliver an excellent service so that your patients and former patients trust you, they are likely to consider you for other problems. Most often the conversation goes as follows:

> Former Patient: "I know you've helped me a lot with being single and dealing with my relationship issues. My friend Susie is going crazy with her teenage son. I think you're terrific but I wasn't sure that you worked with teenagers. Do you? Or do you know someone who does?"

Think of this as a trust factor that preempts almost all other marketing techniques. Sometimes you see the trust factor working in reverse for psychotherapists. Research shows that patients (to the chagrin of psychotherapists) consult their general practitioners (MDs) for psychological problems. In fact, the data have found that 60% of the visits to medical practitioners are for psychologically related problems. The explanation for this finding is that a patient, regardless of the problem, will seek the services of someone they trust.

This research finding can work in our favor. In this mass-marketed, managed care, Internet-bombarded, anonymous world, trusting relationships are becoming increasingly scarce. It is ironic that managed care, with its large volume of patients and diminished time for personal relationships, sets the stage for independent practitioners who are able to spend greater amounts of time with each patient, making them more desirable and therefore more marketable. You, the independent practitioner, generalist or specialist, fill a void created by managed care by providing a needed trusting relationship.

GETTING STARTED

One way to get started thinking about a specialization is to use the broad areas identified by the APA public education research. Their findings identified three areas that the public accepts as open to psychological intervention. These areas are parenting concerns, health issues and workplace stress. We have added one category for "other" as a catchall for other niches that we feel are highly marketable but do not fall within the APA data.

The following subtopics are easy-to-market areas:

• Parenting dilemmas such as ADHD, school problems, step-parenting, child and adolescent parenting concerns, adoption, and learning disabilities
• Health concerns such as weight problems and eating disorders, cancer, serious and chronic illness, smoking, death and dying, memory enhancement, depression, anxiety and panic disorders, infertility, miscarriage, sexual problems, and addictions
• Workplace issues such as career counseling, executive coaching, employee downsizing, worker productivity, sexual harassment, gender discrimination, and team-building skills

In the "other" category we suggest issues such as marital and relationship counseling, gay and lesbian issues, phobias, sport psychology, singles issues, hypnosis, and ethnic-specific therapy.

In determining your niche, consider the following:

• Did you have an internship or work experience that you can use as a specialization?
• Is there an issue or problem that you would like to explore?
• In your therapy practice, what problems have you been most successful in treating?
• When you purchase a psychotherapy book, what topic are you most interested in reading about?
• When you consider attending a continuing education workshop or professional meeting, what catches and holds your attention?
• What hobbies or interests do you have outside of generic psychotherapy?

It is imperative that you feel interested and enthusiastic about your specialty niche because it may require extra learning and focusing to develop both expert skills and a successful marketing program.

EXAMPLES OF SPECIALISTS AND GENERALISTS

Capitalizing on the increasing numbers of older Americans, psychologist Michael Brickey has created a niche market as a longevity coach or therapist. Although he considers himself a generalist, he regards himself as one who is interested in being on the cutting edge of new psychology. He defines this as delivering services in innovative ways. Traditional specialties seemed confining to him, so "I programmed myself to be alert to what would be a specialty that I would love doing and not find confining. I became captivated with the idea of what it takes mentally to live to 150 years of age."

Independent practitioner Brickey notes that in 1995 there were 52,000 centenarians in the United States and that during our lifetime some people will be living to 150. Living mentally healthy will be increasingly important to this population, and he believes that he can set up a specialty that will serve them.[1]

Pamela Chicurel,[2] a clinical nurse specialist in psychiatry nursing, created a niche as a child and adolescent psychotherapist. She developed her interests through a job in a residential treatment center when she first started her training. Her choice of specialization seemed like a natural career for her because she followed her instincts and did what she liked best—she worked with the population she felt most comfortable with. Her enjoyment of working with children and adolescents also comes from her feeling that she relates well to children and understands them. In her role as a child therapist, parents become an essential part of the treatment. Her work takes her into pediatricians' offices and into day-care centers and schools, where she talks with teachers about issues that are relevant to them. In working with pediatricians she often finds that she begins by talking with the nursing staff, a natural association for her. In her general private practice she works with children, adolescents, and adult psychotherapy clients.

Another successful generalist with a niche is Arthur Kovacs (1996), a psychologist who has developed a model that identifies psychotherapists as life span developmental experts. He sees clinicians as being particularly trained to understand individual and family life cycles of development from infancy through old age. He notes that people frequently experience emotional distress at times of transitions. Although these transitions may be normal developmentally, they may still arouse emotional conflicts, anxieties, and depression. Events such as marriage, a birth, the realization that our parents are aging, and our own aging can produce the need to talk with someone who has the competence to help one through these transitions.

A theme that Arthur Kovacs (1996) repeats is that of giving psychology away. This is another term for marketing. As you are "giving it away" you are marketing yourself. You are doing performance advertising. People are seeing you in action, and, if you leave them with a positive impression, they will think of calling you when they have a personal need to see a psychotherapist.

Diana List Cullen,[3] social worker–psychotherapist, seems to have carved out a niche market in the way that Arthur Kovacs suggests. Her practice highlights the steps needed to develop a successful specialization. Concentrating on the relationships between parents and adult children and the difficulties that occur, she advertises her support and discussion groups for individual and couples in free local newspapers, takes out ads, and writes articles in neighborhood "throw-aways."

In her 1991 article Cullen talks about why these relationships go awry and how painful they can be to both the adult children and the parents. She writes about specific issues that have helped clients and about how clients can develop greater respect and trust and build communication bridges. Cullen has developed a non–managed care niche and does pro bono talks at senior centers. She markets to synagogues and physicians, to whom she has written letters and with whom she made personal contact. She is the Immediate Past President of the Metropolitan chapter of the New York State Society for Clinical Social Workers, which contributes to her exposure and marketing. Her practice highlights the steps needed to develop a successful specialization.

REFINING AND DELIVERING YOUR NICHE

After you have identified your specialty you can begin to "refine your niche" to further identify what makes you the best person to deliver this specialized service. Usually, refining a niche can be thought of as distinguishing the service in terms of specialized content, unusual delivery, or outstanding credibility. A creatively delivered niche can change an ordinary topic and change it into an extraordinarily appealing service. Consider the following niche of "singles services" and notice the three innovative and appealing ways that this niche can be refined and delivered.

Specialized Content

The ad "Dating Skills Training" was eye-catching. This singles service captures attention because of its specialized content. Developed by Ann Demarais, psychologist, this service sends patients on a simulated date and then provides them with specific feedback to improve their dating skills (Demarais, 1999). Areas assessed include conversational skills, self-presentation, self-disclosure, sincerity, outlook, showing interest in others' humor, and so on. When interviewed by one of the authors (SH), independent practitioner Demarais stated that her idea for this service was based on her talents as an executive coach and on her belief that single individuals would have the most to gain and the greatest willingness to spend money on a service of this type.

Dating Skills Training has also captured the media's attention and has been featured in national newspapers, magazines, and prime time television.

Unusual Delivery

This was a niche market write up in "Psychotherapy Finances" (Bavonese, 1999). Joe Bavonese, psychologist, offered a Friday night drop in singles support group of $5 per person, advertised in local papers and in the free listing sections of larger papers. His groups quickly grew from 4 to 5 people to 30 to 40 people. Later, he added a once-a-month communication workshop. This unusual delivery of services resulted in patients for his practice and speaking opportunities from the other organizations his singles belonged to.

Outstanding Credibility

Since 1983, Kate Wachs, psychologist, has used her Ph.D. to give credibility to the typically less than credible business of a dating service. In a personal interview, she notes that her professional ethics have made her business more than the usual "take the money and run" service.[4] "If a client is not right, I won't take them, no matter how much money they have." Her well-developed skills have also contributed to her success because she is able to interview, observe, and match her clients more thoroughly than can individuals without her professional training. "Dr. Kate's" credibility and popularity soared even further when she began writing "Love Advice" for America Online (AOL) services.

These individuals are all associated with a specific niche for which they have identified their services as superior. In the first case, there was "real feedback" that would help clients better their self-presentation. In the second case, the distinction was a low-cost opportunity to meet other single people. In the third case, there was the increased credibility of using graduate degrees and knowledge of personality issues to more correctly identify a better mate.

In conclusion we note that

- there are many ways to remain a generalist and still have a niche to market yourself.

- niche marketing and specialization can help you be a successful generalist.
- as new opportunities present themselves, you may find that you have several niches, all of which can be feeders into your general practice.
- in considering a specialization, think about how to distinguish yourself in a community of similar psychotherapists.
- remember to shape your practice according to your interests.
- you may need to learn more before you fill a particular specialization and become identified with it. Your area of interest may require you to take courses, get supervision, find a mentor, or attend a series of conferences.
- an "ordinary" idea or concept delivered in an extraordinary manner will have appeal.

Now that you have identified a niche or specialty, it is time to sharpen your skills so that you are truly marketing a superior product. The next chapter discusses this concept and some of the varied paths our colleagues have traveled in the pursuit of the "gold standard."

NOTES

[1] Personal communication, March 2, 2000.
[2] Personal communication, January 5, 2000.
[3] Personal communication, January 30, 2000.
[4] Personal communication, November 3, 1998.

REFERENCES

Bavonese, J. (1999). *Psychotherapy Finances* (Bonus Report). West Palm Beach, FL: Ridgewood Financial Institute.
Cullen, D. L. (1991, May 20). Don't call me, I won't call you. Upper East Side Resident, p. 202.
Demarais, A. (1999). *Dating skills training.* [Available from A. Demarais, see Appendix]. New York: First Impressions.
Kovacs, A. (1996, May 4). Escaping the industrialization of care: Transforming the structures of practice [workshop]. Los Angeles, CA.
Wachs, K. (1999). *Love Advice.* America Online, Inc.

Chapter 8

Your Path to Success: The Gold Standard

The "gold standard" is the standard against which all is measured. It is derived from the use of gold as measure of monetary worth as compared with any other currency unit. In the United States, the gold standard was the legal weight and quality of gold coins before 1934, and it was the basis of our paper money system. Some of you will also recognize this term because of its current use describing the optimum level of medical treatment. In this chapter, we are using the gold standard to describe the level of excellence needed to successfully market services as an independent psychotherapist.

The well-known small-business marketer Jay Conrad Levinson reminds us that ". . . you understand that you have to offer a quality product or service to be successful. Even the best marketing in the world won't motivate a customer to purchase a poor product or service more than once. In fact, guerrilla marketing can speed the demise of an inferior offering, since people will learn of the shoddiness of that much quicker" (Levinson, 1993, p. 9).

Hans Strupp, a master psychotherapist, notes that technical skills are the "hallmark of the competent psychotherapist" (1999, p. 35). In a recent article, he discusses a study that compared the performance of experienced therapists with the performance of untrained but kind college professors in a therapeutic setting. Strupp reports that the kindly professors soon "ran out of material to talk about," indicating that they were unable to organize, process, and pull together the clinical data in a meaningful manner. Strupp concludes that the excellent therapist has access to a theoretical framework that "may be relatively straightforward but . . . must embody a rationale of what constitutes the 'problem' and what should be done to alleviate it" (p. 35).

BASIC SKILL BUILDING BLOCKS

Excellence in therapeutic skill is most often developed through basic building blocks of advanced educational offerings and through clinical experiences. Examples of such include

- literature review, discussion, and mastery
- professional training audios, videos, and CDs
- continuing education workshops, conferences, and master classes
- part-time postgraduate programs
- weekend immersion courses
- organizational seminars
- study groups and/or peer supervision groups
- dialogues with a mentor, supervisor, or leader
- short-term intensive training programs (typically lasting 1 to 2 weeks)
- on-line (Internet) learning programs
- significant and pivotal life experiences

YOUR SKILL BUILDING GAME PLAN

Gold standard skills result from the continued growth and interconnection of basic skill building blocks. The key is to shape a personal career map for which each educational component or basic building block contributes to the resultant gold standard. As you create your personal map, think in terms of integrating, interconnecting, mastering, and developing your skills.

Similar to winning at chess, each professional move should be made with a clear rationale. Each move has an impact on every other move; the aim is a successful win.

Unfortunately, it is easy to be seduced by offerings that will not contribute to the gold standard. Professional workshops feature a smorgasbord of appealing items that vary from theoretical topics to hands-on skills to sexy tax write-off vacation sprees. Most professionals are flooded with varying opportunities and possibilities. How does the aspiring gold standard therapist reach a winning decision from these many different possibilities?

Consider some of the most appealing brochures with pictures of beach scenes or cruise lines on the cover. Surely, the marketers are selling "relaxation and vacation" as a key part of their offering. They are hoping that you might read this type of brochure in the following manner:

- "Hmm, this looks like a fabulous, appealing beach vacation."
- "Wow, these workshops are offered at many different times, so I can choose whatever vacation period works best for me."
- "That's nice. The courses look pretty interesting, too."

Selecting a workshop offering based on these criteria is fine if your primary goal is vacationing. If your goal is serious gold standard skill building, then you need to choose your workshops more carefully. Reading a sample brochure with skill building in mind might create an internal conversation like this:

- "Hmm, this looks like an in-depth practical offering led by a master therapist that will help me deliver a superior service to my clients."
- "Wow, I'm going to call a few colleagues and check out this presenter and make sure she is both master therapist and superior teacher."
- "This class will build on my previous knowledge and interests. I can see how it will round out my skill base and make me more expert in my field."

If evaluating every brochure sounds onerous to you, then consider creating your skill building game plan with part-time programs that offer a prepared curriculum. Look for courses that are organized (beginner, intermediate, advanced) and offer practical supervised components or videotaped segments. There are often evening or weekend programs in some cities that have the added advantage of offering social contact with colleagues and increased visibility that adds to referral possibilities.

Be wary of single workshops for complex topics (e.g., divorce mediation), because, for most practitioners, they are often too dilute to be confidently integrated into a practice.

FROM PERSONAL EXPERIENCES TO PROFESSIONAL INTERESTS TO THE GOLD STANDARD

Many of the most respected and successful professionals have gone beyond the traditional training possibilities. They have had additional nontraditional experiences that contribute to their gold standard of skill. Some of these additional contributions have come from personal experience, formal research opportunities, self-initiated apprenticeships, and pro bono work, which are often "patched together" in a unique mosaic that results in a gold standard. Here are a sampling of individual paths that have led to the gold standard.

Skill Building from Childhood and Family Milieu

At times one's upbringing and basic life events form a beginning set of lifetime interests and initial skill building abilities on which our future careers are based.

Jane Buckwalter[1] began her child analysis connection long before she ever considered such a career. She remembers being 8 or 9 years old and going to work with her mother, who was a teacher-director at a therapeutic school on Saturdays. This was no ordinary playdate because the children were emotionally disturbed. After this introduction she went on to join the American Friends Service Committee in college, and they assigned her to a volunteer job in a program for autistic children because they thought she was gifted in this area. Throughout her career she has worked with children and families but thought that she should do something more administrative with her social work degree. An evening job in a clinic brought her back to her early connections with disturbed children. She has built her practice based on her early experience and her work experiences and through supervisors, mentors, and a child analytic program. Buckwalter encourages her students and colleagues to consider child therapy work because there is an enormous need but few professionals to fill the gap. Presently, she combines a child and adult practice, supervises, and is the President of the American Mental Health Alliance–New York, which has given her a national referral base. In addition, she does some local public speaking, writes articles, and travels to present at international conferences.

Kate Hays[2] was able to take her lifelong passion for athletics and sports and turn it into a gold standard skill. Supplemented by texts and journal articles, workshops and conferences, informal mentoring, and relationships with experts in the field, Kate Hays became a sports psychologist and started her own organization, "The Performing Edge." As her experience increased, she began writing, first for the general public and then for her profession. Her most recent publication is a book for practitioners on the use of exercise in psychotherapy. Her future plan is to expand her business by extrapolating from sports psychology to other performance areas, specifically with performing artists.

Kate Hays states that her best assets are her solid credentials and her personable interviewing style, both of which have enabled her to do cross-referral and case consultation with sports medicine personnel (orthopedists, physical therapists, nutritionists, and trainers) and directors of performing arts organizations. She keeps both her skills and contacts current in her position as staff sport psychologist for a sports medicine organization where she takes referrals, makes cross-referrals within the organization, provides workshops, and writes for their newsletter.

Dana Ackley[3] is a psychologist who serves as a consultant to businesses. He attributes both his interest and success to customer service principles that he learned in his early years from his family, which ran a small business, and to his brother, who is a highly successful businessman. He notes that these family relationships both helped him learn business fundamentals and allowed him to avoid some of the biases many of our colleagues have about business people. He enjoys providing "first class services that focus on what people want and need, not DSM oriented ideas."

Several years ago, Dana Ackley[4] worked on the Virginia Marketing Project through the Virginia Psychology Association. He notes that "doing the literature review helped me rediscover my (and our) value, learning that action overcomes depression, recognizing the hopelessness of fighting managed care and replacing it with a 'better' third party system, and learning about the needs and opportunities for us in the business world." In this professional capacity, he learned more about working with businesses and rounded out his personal experiences by reading and taking workshops. Dana Ackley stays current through his work with the local Chamber of Commerce, Kiwanis Club, and United Way.

Ron Fox, psychologist, gave his old-time business interests a new twist with a telephone coaching service for business executives, particularly those in family businesses. His service addresses major problems that can arise when family members have differences about their business, when family members cannot separate family and business issues, and when family members experience difficulty in focusing on the most important issues that confront their business and their family.

The basis for Ron Fox's interests was his own family experience.

I was raised in a family business and had management/supervisory/ responsibilities at a very young age and a father who was very supportive in the crunch. Once he told me to work in our shipping department to find out who was stealing from us and fire them. I was afraid to do that. The kind of people who worked there were transient, combative and would not shrink from beating up the boss' son. I resisted dad's request saying I was just a kid (age 16, barely). He said, 'I don't have anyone else to help. You just do your best. We never kicked anyone out of the family because they did their best and failed!' A very powerful message, indeed.[5]

These early personal experiences came into play when then as a university dean Ron Fox[6] was asked by business executives to help out with problems they were having with other executives. He addressed their concerns and supplemented his experiential knowledge base with courses from experts on related topics and mentoring by a leading psychology process consultant . He also notes that there are many skills as a therapist (and particularly as a family therapist) that he could transfer to help him further develop his gold standard of skills as a business consultant.

Skill Building From Crisis

Crises of trauma and loss are devastating events. For some psychotherapists, the process of coping and recovery from these ordeals sets the stage for gold standard skills.

Psychologist Laurie Kolt's[7] personal battle with infertility and miscarriages forms the basis for her professional development as an infertility expert. She notes that she supplemented her personal experience by way of a thorough literature review at the local medical library, cross-referencing psychology, psychotherapy, and infertility. There were about 300 articles at the time, and she put them into a three-ring binder and organized them using different colored magic markers for different issues. For example, she separated out the information that was relevant for medical doctors, men's infertility issues, women's infertility issues, and couple's issues. This system enabled her to note the many trends that were key to program development, interacting with referral sources and the public.

After digesting the literature, she consulted with a leading psychologist to refine her ideas and and help her clarify the psychological issues involved in working with infertile clients. She also joined professional groups that would further her insight into the "culture" of infertility, particularly from a client's point of view.

Donna Harris,[8] a social worker-psychoanalyst who specializes in trauma and substance abuse, grew up in a household with a famous jazz musician father and a creative fashion designer mother. At age 10, when her family moved to Brussels, Belgium, she dealt with the traumatic impact of leaving everything she knew. She had to learn French and Flemish and be a black American child in a white European culture. "Cars would stop and people would stare at us on the street because they never saw American black people. I was always pointed out as different."[9] It was not until she went to social work school for her second masters degree (she also has a masters degree in psychology) that she began to fully accept her connection to addictions and being a caretaker, having seen the effect of drug and alcohol abuse within her family. She attended workshops, seminars, and programs on substance abuse. Prior to analytic training she worked in the field of chemical dependency and mentally ill chemical abusers (MICA) for 6 years and continued for 3 more years working with chemically dependent women with histories of sexual abuse. "At the last two jobs I was involved with program development, supervision and treatment, so I learned a lot."[10] In addition to her private practice and faculty position, she has developed with Susan Rios, a social worker and psychoanalyst, a new business venture: the New York Association of Trauma Psychotherapists.

Ellen McGrath[11] is a psychologist who spent a good deal of her young adulthood battling depression.

> We didn't have much money growing up. My parents separated when I was 10 and divorced when I was 13, and my father died with my 14-year-old brother in a violent car crash when I was 17. We had separating, divorce, death, all those things happen in 7 years, and we had no money and no educational opportunities, nothing. . . . my mother was not strong, not available to me in many ways. . . . My father had an identical twin brother who shot himself in the head with a shotgun. And he had a sister who also committed suicide. I had (the vulnerability) because I had overwhelming losses.

Ellen McGrath is open about these painful experiences and uses them as a tool in her work with depressed patients. "The number one lesson I've learned is to connect to people and to remove as many obstacles to connecting as I can. I've had centuries of personal psychotherapy that have taught me the life skills that I was missing. I understand that my depression and pain is what gives me the cutting edge in helping people and in knowing what they are experiencing."[12] In her efforts to conquer her problem, she explored long-term intensive interpersonal psychotherapy with several different clinicians, cognitive therapy with an emphasis on disputing skills and cognitive restructuring, psychotherapy with a focus on narcissistic family disorders, eye movement desensitization and reprocessing (EMDR), and psychotropic medications.

Throughout her professional career, she has continued to gather and master the research on the latest medical, psychological, traditional psychopharmacological, and alternative medical (e.g., St. John's wort) interventions. She has offered to integrate and publish the existing research and clinical materials and became the chair of a task force on women and depression for the APA. Following this, she translated her research experience into two mass market books on depression. These materials, along with her own personal examples, formed the basis for keynote speeches and workshops delivered throughout the country.

Alice Chang is a psychologist whose interests became more focused after her own experience with cancer. Although her training program included work with cancer patients, it was only after her cancer experience that work

> Just got more focused and intense because of my sense of needing to do something more now!!!—which as you know is not an uncommon feeling among survivors . . . . I learned almost everything 'flying by the seat of my pants.' I talk with psychologists, physicians, oncologists, internists, radiologists, surgeons at every opportunity and I check the Internet sites for further help. In addition, I talk with current and past cancer patients as I meet them, wherever I meet them. I am a self-trained medical psychological consultant person since I started long before any of this was in vogue . . . by creating liaisons with individuals' care givers along the way. I find folks who need my services whom I respect.
> I have attended some CE classes on medically related disorders and given a lot of thought to how the implications fit with my work, etc. And, I give a lot of talks these days, which means that I get a lot of interesting feedback. I read what I can, when I can.[13]

Alice Chang's experiences culminated in the formation of a nonprofit organization, the Academy for Cancer Wellness, which helps people recognize each other as cancer survivors or champions. She recently completed a book and a play that describe her cancer experience from the perspective of both a patient and a psychologist.

Additional Postgraduate Education, Training, or Clinical Experience

Sometimes actual work experiences serve to sharpen skills and help professionals hone in on needs that are traditionally overlooked or inadequately served.

Rosemary Lavinski, a dynamically trained social worker, saw the need for career counseling for some of her patients. When referrals to career coaches had disappointing results, she decided to expand her practice and her skills into this specialty area.[14]

"Since I had an interest in folks' work life I pursued career counseling." A one-year-post-masters' training in career counseling along with supervision from a prominent career coach yielded her gold standard skills, which she markets informally through word of mouth and formally through a brochure, newsletter, Web page, postcard ad, and targeted mailing list.[15]

Leslie Malin is a social worker–psychotherapist who combined her knowledge of therapy and experience in hospitals to become a successful therapist, consultant, speaker, and entrepreneur—founder of

Management by Design, a human resources assessment and development firm.

In her early days as an inpatient social worker in a psychiatric hospital, Malin did individual, family, and group therapy. Through her work, she developed an understanding of family and group dynamics and began to give lectures at grand rounds and do inservice training with the staff. She enlarged on her already formidable skills as a presenter when she became the clinical director of a mental health program for teens and families and then joined and spoke at community boards.[16]

Malin presents workshops and retreats for organizations that want to bring a new vitality and spirit into the workplace. She also offers life journey workshops for individuals.

In a new and innovative venture, Malin developed (with a graphics designer) "Earth Medicine," a business to business greeting card company that combines beautiful images with messages of concern and meaning. For Malin, "Everything I do is a form of therapy and healing."[17] Marketing on the Internet and through e-mail newsletters (e-zine) and joining formal networking groups have been successful for her.

Psychologist Lenore Walker developed her skills with battered women and abuse victims from working directly with her clients. Initially, she tried to apply what she knew about trauma and abuse to the treatment but found it to be only minimally helpful. She improvised and applied feminist psychological principles to her work and continuously evaluated the impact of her approach on the client. She then designed a research program on a more diverse sample of women to assess whether her approach was effective. It was. She took her ideas and the issues a step further—to legislators and congressional leaders who in turn directed her to the National Institute of Mental Health (NIMH), which was dealing with violence and behavior issues. She was asked to meet with NIMH staff and congressional representatives to report on her innovative approach. This began her work in applying psychological data to public policy makers.[18]

In taking her gold standard one step further, she then attended several practical continuing education workshops on how to be an expert witness, and over the years continued to read materials on this topic. In the mid to late 1980s she was appointed to the APA Committee on Legal Issues and became more familiar with the APA Amicus Brief program. She then began working with outstanding lawyers who helped her to apply her psychological knowledge of battered women to legal cases. Lenore Walker's name appeared in several of the early defining cases that allowed battered woman syndrome testimony to be admitted on behalf of battered women who said that they killed their abusive partner in self-defense.

Publication of journal articles and books brought more publicity and established her as an expert this unusual niche.

Gold Standard Through Multiple Credentials

At times, a unique gold standard can be created from a work history that has multiple professional credentials. Consider the following "gold standard" psychotherapists.

Dolores Walker was an attorney for 10 years prior to her return to school to obtain her masters degree in social work. She trained as a mediator at the same time she completed her masters degree.

> I discovered that the two groups who specialize in mediation are mental health professionals and attorneys. This meant that I was uniquely qualified. There are only four or five mediators in New York City who are both attorneys and psychotherapists. In my marketing, I emphasized my dual expertise. I co-authored an article for the Big-Apple Parents newspaper and arranged for a seminar which was listed next to my byline. I sent an Academy of Family Mediators' brochure explaining mediation, a separate brochure describing my background, and a personalized letter to other psychotherapists in the therapy suite, in the office building, friends, colleagues, etc., and I continued to send letters to my ever-growing mailing list, including notes with holiday cards, to everyone I knew. I joined many organizations, advertised in niche publications, and, with a colleague, offered seminars through the Learning Annex and New York University's continuing education program. After five years in the field, I became a board member of the Family & Divorce Mediation Council of greater New York.[19]

Michael Enright's general psychology practice is located in Jackson Hole, Wyoming. As a practitioner in a rural area and in an office in a building that he part owns with two pediatricians, a family physician, a dermatologist, and a surgeon, Enright often found himself in the position of informally and formally suggesting psychotropic medication to his colleagues. His experiences and the needs of his colleagues and patients led him to be a long time advocate for prescription privileges and has taken the personal responsibility of getting this for himself before organized psychology voiced any interest or support for this skill. He has already completed his prescriptive training, is a Registered Nurse, and is now in the process of advanced nurse training so that he can prescribe medication as a psychiatric nurse.[20]

Patricia Pimental built her neuropsychology skills with her internships, practicas, postdoctoral training, workshops, research, writing, and her dissertation, all of which resulted in her developing a new right hemisphere screening instrument.[21] For her rehabilitation work, she had already had a masters degree in speech pathology, worked as a speech-language pathologist for 8 years, and learned to communicate in sign language. To increase her knowledge in behavioral medicine-health, mind-body medicine, and pain management she attended special workshops, seminars, and hypnosis training with leading experts in the field.

Her skills stay current through informal conversations and case consultations with colleagues in the medical community. With her office in close proximity to about 15 medical doctors who from time to time "drop by and plop on my chair and talk for a few minutes . . . stress relief. I've got chocolates on my desk and a running fountain and dim lamp lighting, like home, stress reducing."[22]

These various examples can provide you with the understanding of the many different paths open to mental health professionals in achieving a gold standard of expertise. We encourage you to find your path of gold standard skill development, bearing in mind the adage that "knowledge is power." In chapter 9 we will show you how to use your skills as a valuable offering to another professional's businesses or practice. Developing gold standard skills is a solid beginning on your path to success.

NOTES

[1] Personal communication, January 3, 2000.
[2] Personal communication, April 5, 1999.
[3] Personal communication, March 1, 1999.
[4] Personal communication, May 1, 1999.
[5] Personal communication, April 5, 1999.
[6] Personal communication, April 5, 1999.
[7] Personal communication, January 7, 1999.
[8] Personal communication, January 13, 2000.
[9] Personal communication, January 13, 2000.
[10] Personal communication, January 13, 2000.
[11] Personal communication, May 15, 2000.
[12] Personal communication, May 15, 2000.
[13] Personal communication, January 10, 2000.
[14] Personal communication, December 11, 1999.
[15] Personal communication, December 11, 1999.
[16] Personal communication, January 13, 2000.
[17] Personal communication, January 13, 2000.
[18] Personal communication, April 16, 1999.
[19] Personal communication, December 8, 1999.
[20] Personal communication, March 30, 1999.
[21] Personal communication, April 14, 1999.
[22] Personal communication, April 14, 1999.

REFERENCES

Levinson, J. C. (1993). *Guerrilla marketing.* New York: Houghton Mifflin Co.
Strupp, H. (1999, Winter). In Three things that make my psychotherapy effective. Division of *Psychotherapy Bulletin, 34,* 22–36.

Chapter 9

Value-Added Services: Why Other Professionals Need Psychotherapists

The business of psychotherapy is based on referrals. Asking colleagues to send you new patients is the most frequent method of generating referrals. Unfortunately, there is little certainty and a great deal of anxiety to this method.

Imagine if things were different. Imagine that your services are in continuous demand. Imagine that your services are thought of as a business asset. This can happen as you apply your psychotherapy skills to improving the business of other professions. In this approach, adding the services of a psychotherapist gives a value-added feature to the other profession, helping it draw and maintain clients. You become an essential part of their marketing plan. You become part of their product line. Like the business-to-business telephone directories, your psychotherapy business can add a new dimension to another to another type of business. You become a value-added service to the other profession or business. Value-added service differs from simply getting referrals. Consider the following examples:

Referral: A cardiologist suggests that a patient see you when the topic of a high-stress job comes up.

Value-Added Service: You deliver a stress reduction workshop once a month at a local cardiologist's office. The cardiologist describes this to all new patients as part of the program.

Referral: A client at a beauty salon confides her age-related sexual concerns to her beautician. The beautician gives the client your name and number and suggests that you can be helpful with these concerns.

Value-Added Service: The beauty salon offers a makeover workshop for midlife women. You address the concept of self-confidence and sexual attraction. The salon offers this workshop to all of its customers and posts the upcoming event in the display window.

The examples of psychotherapy as a value-added service are endless and can include any creative connection with other professions or businesses in your community where your service adds to their business. Other examples of psychotherapy as a value-added service include relationships with pediatricians, dentists, oncologists, clergy, and funeral directors. Although in some cases some new information or experience regarding the specifics of the other profession may be valuable, usually no extensive training or certification is necessary. Most of you will already have the fundamental education, training, and experience necessary.

So now you may wonder "what's in it for you?" Even if you think you can help another profession, how is this going to help you? The answer is "exposure." While you are enhancing the business of the other professional you are advertising, marketing, and exposing yourself to a specific group of persons who are very likely to think of you when they think of seeing a psychotherapist. With your volunteer time you are basically buying advertising for yourself. Think of this as a personal infomercial. You will be given the arena to show your wares, yet you are not "selling," and the persons receiving your services are not "buying," at least not at the moment. In their minds you will become their expert, and they will come to like and trust your knowledge. You certainly must leave them with fact sheets on the topics that you cover and brochures, outlines, or other appropriate items that should have your name and phone number included.

The difficulty that you may face in using these ideas may again be more a function of your own insecurities and self-esteem as a value-added service for other professionals, rather than from any real problems inherent in this venture. Just like the issues regarding money and the ability to ask for adequate income and payment, thinking of yourself as a value-added component for the local pediatrician may just feel too ambitious for you. It may sound too egotistical to you. You may want to talk with other psychotherapists who offer services in this manner or look around at those professional offices where a psychotherapist is included. What is the reputation of that office and psychotherapist? Most probably it is quite high. Think about whether any ambivalent feelings about doing this type of service have more to do with your low self-confidence than with a real negative professional reason.

Keep in mind that we are not creating a cookie cutter model of "the" perfect approach to any of the following examples. As you read this chapter, do stop to imagine yourself in the situation with each specific professional. There will be some examples that you most likely will have absolutely no interest in pursuing. Your interest may be awakened by one of our examples, or one of our examples may spur you on to think of your own unique possibilities. Keep in mind that psychotherapists do not have one personality, we come in all styles, and you can certainly fit your style into this concept. If you are socially confident and already take an active role in community or organization groups, this may appear easier. If you are shy you can still use this concept. You may want to pursue written value-added services, such as fact sheets, contributions to business newsletters, and Web sites, or you may want to ease the path by preparing more materials, preparing a letter of introduction, or creating a packet of information about yourself, or a combination of these.

In this chapter, we will sample several areas where clinicians have contributed a "value-added" feature to other businesses and, in so doing, have created an ongoing demand for their services. There are wonderful, interesting, and lucrative opportunities right around you in your own community and perhaps in your own office building. You do not need extensive extra training, you do not need a new degree or certification, and clearly you do not need an MBA. Realize that you frequently help out your individual patients in their career or business in the course of psychotherapy. You probably have been doing this on a one-to-one basis for years without identifying it. Now we are asking you to look around in your own community, at your acquaintances, and at your office building colleagues. We want you to open your eyes to the practice opportunities right before you.

CLERGY

Religious institutions need members. Although we usually do not think of a religious organization as a business, in fact, it is. Churches and synagogues depend on membership fees and donations to maintain their buildings, pay salaries, and provide services. Liaisons with clergy can range from assisting the clergy in dealing with members of their congregation who are in need of mental health services as well as working together in prevention programs for the community. Although some clergy are trained in pastoral counseling, they usually prefer to not have a long-term psychotherapy situation with one of their congregants. Consider volunteering to lead a lecture or series that is psychological in nature, such as Communicating with your Teen, Drug Information for Parents and Teens, Prenuptial Couples Groups, or Bereavement Groups. Again, this is a win, win, win situation. The synagogue or church will attract and retain congregants who desire the relevant and helpful programs that you can offer. The congregants win because their needs are being served. You win because you have established a forum for yourself in your own community that also exposes you to potential patients. Additionally, the clergyperson is more likely to refer a congregant to you once he or she becomes comfortable with your work.

Notice, you do not need to get an added certificate in theology or take any specific continuing education courses to be capable of offering a very beneficial service to these persons. Your knowledge, education, and training are already sufficient to allow you to be seen as a professional who brings value-added information and service to the congregation. Your approach, whether reserved or gregarious, will still be heard by the clergy whom you approach with your idea. To help with your initial communication with the clergy, have a prepared outline of the service(s) that you are ready to volunteer to the congregation. You may want to have outlines on one or more topics. Make an appointment for a meeting and propose your concept of volunteering for the specific service. Although you will want to remain flexible to the needs and schedules of the church or synagogue, you must begin with a plan. Your plan will set the stage and deliver the concept that you can provide a service that will be beneficial to the congregation and why.

FUNERAL HOMES

Eric Farwell, a funeral director in La Jolla, California, is one of the new breed of funeral directors concerned with "after care."[1] This care addresses the bereavement process for the entire family. More expanded services are also possible. The Frank E. Campbell Funeral Chapel in New York City offers monthly seminars on timely topics such as "Holiday Blues Without a Loved One." New funeral director professionals are trained in knowing how to extend bereavement counseling to the family regarding their loss. In cases of traumatic deaths or severe or prolonged bereavement, these funeral directors enhance their offering by being able to refer clients to therapists in the community. This improves the services offered by the mortuary and creates a reputation within the community of a "caring mortuary facility."

If you are interested in developing a relationship with funeral directors in your area, you will be most successful with those who already offer "after care." Mr. Farwell noted that the buzzword to use in a cold call to a mortuary is to ask if they provide "after care."[2] If there is no response to this term, try another mortuary. Again, have a concept of the type of service that you will be interested in providing. You may want to offer a lecture or a series of lectures on bereavement, or you may want to focus on specific issues such as loss of a spouse or a child or a topic such as suicide or violence. Meet with the funeral director and propose your ideas and ask about his or her own needs for this service.

Do not worry about your lack of knowledge about this profession; most people outside the profession are very uninformed about the funeral business. This is something that the newer funeral directors are aware of and want to help change. The fear, avoidance, and denial of death in our society is very strong and is associated with the funeral business. However, death does come to everyone, and it is something that every person deals with at different times in life. It is a business that does indeed have a need for services that we can provide.

Make your call to your local funeral directors. Have your thoughts prepared regarding the services you can provide. Gather some information to create a handout with your name and phone number.

DENTISTS

Most psychotherapists overlook the fact that many dental problems have a psychological basis. Dental symptoms such as temporal mandibular disease (TMD, previously known as TMJ), bruxism, dental phobia, dental anxiety, and bulimia are all mental health issues that manifest themselves in dental problems and disease. Dentists are usually quite aware of this, and their journals and workshops speak to this reality. Truth is, most of them are uncomfortable and uncertain about how to talk with a dental patient about these symptoms. Many people with dental anxiety or phobia are experiencing primitive feelings that occur because they need to lie in a helpless, supine position while the dentist works in their mouth, often causing considerable discomfort. Patients' anxieties and discomfort are apparent to dentists, although they usually do not know how to address them.

Other dental concerns relevant to psychotherapists include feelings about tooth loss and the need for prosthodontic replacement (false teeth) as related to issues of self-esteem and body image. Begin with your own dentist. Plan an outline for a talk on any of the previous topics and volunteer to have this take place in the dental office waiting room. Explain how you can develop a talk or discussion group on any topic that appears to be a current issue for the dentist.

You can connect with a local pediatric dentist and give a talk on thumb-sucking and pacifier use in infants, toddlers, and preschoolers. Delivering the talk at the dentist's office makes you a value-added service that the dentist is offering the patients. The patients, new parents, usually are hungry for information on these topics. The dentist may inform them that their child must give up the thumb sucking or pacifier but may not know how to educate them about how to go about this weaning process with their child. The dentist may not be comfortable with dealing with parents' anxieties about the transitions in their child's life. You are the trained professional who can make these transitions easier for the new parents, the child, and the dentist.

Finally, because most good dental work is prevention, dentists are frustrated that they cannot serve some patients sooner. This collaboration is a clear situation whereby psychotherapists can help to bring emotionally reluctant patients into the dentist's office and consult with dentists on identification and assessment of a variety of patient problems.

PEDIATRICIANS

Another profession in which psychotherapists have a very obvious value-added presence is pediatrics.

Parents usually choose pediatricians on word-of-mouth recommendations and so strong is the power of these recommendations that parents will often choose their health plan depending on whether the pediatrician they prefer is a member. Clinicians can be part of this service (whether part of or independent from the group) and add a major new dimension to the satisfaction of parents. Therapists can conduct ongoing group discussions for parents of newborns or on other specific topics, such as toilet training, the "terrible 2s," and developmental patterns that are usually such anxiety to parents. Parenting skills can be part of an ongoing educational program. Brochures or information fact sheets can be made available (with your name, address, and phone imprinted on them). Consultation for more specific problems (colicky babies or "difficult" children) can be conducted so that parents feel more comfort and less stigma in talking with a psychotherapist than they would if they needed to find their own therapist. The presence of the psychotherapist as part of the services available from a pediatrician's office adds to that positive word of mouth information and makes this type of office more popular with parents.

ONCOLOGISTS

Now that there is government funding for the National Center for Complementary and Alternative Medicine (NCCAM) both patients and oncologists have become more interested in the mind and body connection. This sanction, along with two pieces of powerful research— one on the effect of hypnosis and relaxation on controlling the side effects of chemotherapy and the second on the positive impact of support groups on cancer patients—have helped psychotherapists to open the doors to oncologists' offices. The oncologists who can offer psychotherapy services are attractive to anxious and frightened cancer patients and their families. Possible offerings include waiting room workshops on stress management, anxiety reduction, coping with chemotherapy, and family communication. Workshops can be offered for cancer patients or their partners, or both. Psychotherapy services add a valuable and distinctive feature to a traditional oncology practice.

WEB SITES

For any topic that you may address, there is a Web site. Health Web sites are very popular on every topic from information through advice on every possible health-related issue. Most health sites also include emotionally based issues as well as topics that are singularly related to stress, depression, anxiety, relationships, and children. Some sites focus totally on relationships. These sites continue to post new information each day and are always searching for more information and new professionals to contribute to their site. The goal is to draw clients to the site, and you, the psychology expert, can help them do this.

For example, December provides an opportunity for an information piece on holiday stress. Such pieces typically appear with several identifying pieces of information, including your photo, brief biography, address, and personal Web site or e-mail address, or both.

You are bringing value-added service to the Web site a by contributing your information. The Web site owners show their visitors that they have a professional contributing information on their subject of interest. The visitors to the site who read your information have gained this knowledge, so they also are in a win situation. What is your win situation here? Usually not the pay, because this is typically an unpaid contribution. Rather, you have gained exposure and "free" advertising regarding who you are, where you practice, and what you know about this specific topic. Visitors to the site may think of contacting you if they want more information or psychotherapy regarding the issue.

Psychotherapists can be outstanding business builders for almost every professional. If you are trying to fill your appointment book, look to your professional neighbors and identify ways to increase their business. Your dentist, physician, tax preparer, and hairdresser all face problems in owning, managing, and servicing their businesses. If you can assist them and contribute information to their clients, you will be included in a new venture and gain needed exposure for yourself. Truly a win-win situation for psychotherapists who are business builders because they wind up maximizing their own businesses, too.

NOTES

[1] Personal communication, February 13, 1999.
[2] Personal communication, February 13, 1999.

Chapter 10

It Is Moral to Market

M arketing is everything you do to promote yourself and your psychotherapy practice. Marketing is an alien concept to most psychotherapists because it raises anxieties about professionalism and self-promotion. In the past, most clinicians felt that if they were "good" therapists, well-spoken and well-liked, referrals would simply come their way. Marketing seemed too grandiose, overtly ambitious, and downright sleazy.

WHY MARKETING IS IMPORTANT FOR PSYCHOTHERAPISTS

Advice from Professional Marketers

Marketing is very much an appropriate activity for the small business person and even offers several advantages when compared with large corporate marketing. Jay Conrad Levinson (1993), author of *Guerrilla Marketing,* notes that the "little guy" does not "have a body of rules to follow, a committee to answer to, a set structure to follow. You're a guerrilla. You are the organization. You answer to yourself. You make the rules and you break the rules. And that means you get to be amazing, outrageous, surprising, unpredictable, brilliant, and quick" (p. 19).

Kim Ricketts,[1] president of Strategease consulting firm, believes that psychotherapists should market their services. She notes that prior to the era of managed care, therapists could enjoy a steady flow of patients, both with and without insurance reimbursement, and were paid a fair fee for their services. This is no longer possible. Without a successful marketing program, a psychotherapist could easily work more than 60 hours a week for 50% of the previous revenue. Kim notes that the "best ways for psychotherapists to market themselves begins with thinking outside of the box when it comes to the profile of their potential patient. For instance, a psychotherapist specializing in children may consider their patient profile to be the child and family members."[2]

Rhea Farberman, Director of Public Affairs for the APA, agrees that marketing is important for mental health professionals. She notes that "clients are consumers and consumers make buying decisions based on their knowledge/perceptions of the products—all gained by exposure to marketing. . . . Consumers will not understand the value of what you do unless you actively seek to educate them."[3]

The APA is a generally conservative organization very concerned with the ethical standards of their members. In 1994 they launched a public education campaign designed to educate and inform the public about when and how to seek help for emotional problems (American Psychological Association [APA], 1994). The initial stage of the project was a research survey of 1001 men and women who were health care decision makers for their family. There were two findings from this study that are pertinent to the development of your direct pay practice.

1. Eighty-four percent of the consumers understood the link between mental health and physical health.
2. Despite this understood connection, consumers were likely to consult mental health professionals only for traditional problems and serious mental health issues.

The APA survey indicated that the public has already created links of understanding that psychotherapy can help with depression, suicide, and drug or alcohol dependency (APA, 1994). We now need to expand those links so the public also understands that psychotherapy can also help when their children are having problems, they are having stress at work, there are marital problems or divorce, there is serious or chronic disease in a family member, there are infertility problems, or there has been a death in the family.

This information may make it easier for you to see how marketing as public information is for the public good, as well as being in your own professional interest. Marketing in the form of public education is a valuable and ethical endeavor.

Advice From Psychotherapist Marketers

According to Leslie Davenport,[4] social worker and marketing consultant, ". . . client referrals are the lifeblood of any private practice of psychotherapy."

> Without them, we have no business and, therefore, no ability to do the work that we love and have spent years training to do. Somehow we tend to shrink away from the idea that we must attract "customers" (i.e., referrals) through marketing strategies. Perhaps we believe that this trivializes our noble work. Or, we might think that if we are truly good at what we do then the referrals will naturally come our way. This is an unrealistic but common myth among psychotherapists. . . . Some psychotherapists are inhibited about promoting themselves because they fear failure and initially lack self-assurance in their skills. Telling the world about yourself can be a bit scary. What if one doesn't live up to others' expectations? It is important to remember, however, that we are not selling ourselves but rather what we do, our knowledge and clinical expertise as well as the services we offer.[5]

In order to succeed in a direct pay practice you need to seriously consider marketing yourself to become more visible. Rick Marek, a marriage counselor, is very clear about this: "They will forget you! Learn from Coke® and Pepsi®. They continually keep their name in front of us."[6]

"I will market the rest of my professional career," says Rosemary Lavinski, social worker, career counselor, and psychotherapist.[7] "Perhaps the biggest mistake professionals make is to feel they are so well known they can 'coast'."

Kate Hays,[8] sports psychologist, described her marketing efforts after moving from New Hampshire to Toronto and wanting to expand her work with sports to other performance areas, such as performing arts. She noted that in New Hampshire it was quite easy to be known for her work and described it as a "small pond." However, Toronto was a large city in a new country. She described her early marketing efforts in Toronto as a "full time job as I'm really interested in increasing the proportion of my practice devoted to performance issues. There seems to be a very large potential market (major teams, a number of universities, and a variety of cultural organizations)."[9]

MARKETING FEARS AND WORRIES

There are two key reasons that therapists avoid marketing. First, many of us are still unresolved regarding the ethics and professionalism of marketing. Second, even if we are resolved on the first issue, we mistakenly assume that marketing is too expensive.

Worry Number One: Marketing, Professionalism and Ethics

Addressing the first issue, we note that in recent years most professional organizations have opened the door to the idea of clinicians "advertising" to the public. Such advertising tends to be educational. Organizations usually include a strong public service component that offers psychological information. Following this information there can be the name(s) or organization from which one may get more material or direct help.

Consider a recent advertisement produced by the APA: The ad shows a man's worried face. The major caption reads "Ever since the big lay-off, weird things started happening to me. I couldn't sleep or eat. I'd scream at my kids for the littlest things. My job had become a living nightmare (Practice Directorate Public Education Program, American Psychological Association, 1996)." The informational piece then goes on to describe workplace stress and how a psychologist was helpful. The tag line at the bottom of the ad is "Talk to someone who can help," and an 800 number and Web site address are offered for further information.

There are many topics that lend themselves to public information giveaways that you are familiar with and that the public is open to learning about. Examples include information pertaining to the emotional effects of natural disasters, divorce and separation, and chronic illness and why certain emotional conditions occur and what treatments are most viable. Common symptoms such as anxiety, depression, and stress; everyday problems of anger and intimacy; communication skills; and parenting are also topics with universal appeal. Recently, the aging members of the baby boom generation have been open to information about maintaining their physical and mental health, and they are learning that the two are interrelated. Psychological information delivered through media messages has made the mind and body connection a popular household concept.

It is important to recognize that the audience (the public) is there and will listen to whatever information they hear. As ethical and professional psychotherapists, it is part of our responsibility to help educate the public regarding psychological information and services. If they do not hear it from us, they will be open to misinformation from less professional sources.

To reduce your own ethical concern regarding your marketing efforts, follow the lead of professional associations that encourage professional marketing practices to the public. The public education/marketing ad shown in Figure 10.1 appeared in a small New York City parenting newspaper. Independent practitioner Karen Zager and one of the authors (SH) decided to do a series of public education ads as a part of a marketing strategy for a program called "parenting solutions."

Worry Number Two: The Expense of Marketing

The second reason many psychotherapists avoid marketing is the worry that marketing will be too expensive. If this is true for you, it probably means that you have confused the process of marketing with the specifics of advertising. Advertising is only one type of marketing, and, indeed, it can be costly. Marketing, on the other hand, includes many inexpensive communications including your business cards and stationery, the location and hours of your office, brochures that you distribute, seminars and workshops that your offer, public relations, follow-up letters, and, of course, paid advertising. Some of these expenses do not involve monetary outlay but investments of time. Yes, time is money, but time may be the most you have to invest for your effective marketing campaign. Remember how much time you spent completing managed care forms, waiting on hold on the phone, and complaining to your spouse or colleagues about abuses you have endured from managed care reviewers. Those were time investments with no payoff. Now you can use those hours productively and build your managed care–free practice.

It is important to remember that marketing can be both low cost and effective. Public education and informational marketing is one of the easiest and most palatable ways of self-marketing. This is a "soft sell" marketing that aims at self-promotion through public education. It rests on the assumption that a successful public education campaign about anything (be it pesticides or vitamins) will increase the demand in consumers' behavior and cause them to pursue a product that is perceived to be valuable. Examples of low-cost effective marketing follow:

FIGURE 10.1   An example of a public information giveaway advertisement.

- Judith Kottick and Dolores Walker, both social worker psychotherapists, wrote an article for the *Big Apple Parents' Paper* about divorce mediation that included information about the issues related to divorce and an outline of steps and quotes from clients as well as other psychotherapists (Kottick & Walker, 1992).
- Dana Ackley, psychologist, noted that "I got myself in the paper last fall—they did a great article about my book with my picture on the front page of the Sunday business section." His article related to consulting to businesses.[10]
- Adrienne Lampert, social worker, answers questions to readers in a business-oriented local newspaper. Topics in her "Working It Out" column are intended to help business managers "gain new insights in ways of handling 'people problems'" (Lampert, 1994).
- Patricia Pimental,[11] neuropsychologist, works as a Red Cross volunteer on the disaster mental health network and "worked for six hours at a bus-train disaster. . . . without expecting this, I had an interview on local NBC TV . . . this often happens at disasters. You help people and get unexpected (but welcome at no cost) media coverage."

So now it is time for you to begin to think of marketing your service. As a person with a small business, you have the flexibility to choose several different marketing strategies as you see fit. You now know that it is considered moral to market and that you can present yourself and your services in an ethical and professional manner. You also know that there is a minimum in out-of-pocket costs. In chapter 11 you will learn more about specific marketing techniques that will further build your successful independent psychotherapy practice.

NOTES

[1] Personal communication, March 31, 1999.
[2] Personal communication, March 3, 1999.
[3] Personal communication, March 3, 1999.
[4] Personal communication, January 4, 2000.
[5] Personal communication, January 4, 2000.
[6] Personal communication, January 11, 2000.
[7] Personal communication, December 11, 1999.
[8] Personal communication, April 5, 1999.
[9] Personal communication, April 5, 1999.
[10] Personal communication, May 1, 1999.
[11] Personal communication, April 14, 1999.

REFERENCES

American Psychological Association. (1994). *Talk to Someone Who Can Help, Campaign Kit.* Washington, DC: Author.
Kottick, J., & Walker, D. (1992). A referee? *The Big Apple Parent's Paper,* Spring, p. 12.
Lampert, A. (1994). [Column]. Working it out. *Brooklyn Progress.*
Levinson, J. C. (1993). *Guerrilla marketing.* New York: Houghton Mifflin.

Part IV

Basic Tools of the Trade

Chapter 11

Stationery and Business Cards

This chapter will review the basic marketing tools you can use to promote your private practice. How can you get the most mileage out of professional stationery and business cards? We invite you to consider ways you can make these most basic instruments more unique and memorable.

STATIONERY

Stationery is the most basic tool of all. Stationery will contain professional identifying information. In addition to the most obvious suggestion of using a professional quality paper, we also suggest that you consider using your stationery to highlight special features about your practice, described later in the section on business cards. Because stationery should have plenty of space for text, it will usually only carry the basic identifying information and a logo.

The basic information you should have on stationery is your name, degree, title, address, and phone number. Some states require that you include your license number on all stationery and business cards. If you are incorporated, this must appear on your stationery.

You must give thought to whether you want to include your fax number or e-mail address. Most psychotherapists prefer that their patients have only one mode of contact—the telephone. If there are fax numbers and e-mail addresses listed, patients may feel free to contact you through these other means. They may cancel an appointment by e-mail, not knowing that perhaps you do not check your e-mail every day. They may fax you pages of their journal for your review. You may not appreciate this. It is usual to have only information that you want your patients to have on your stationery and business cards. If you choose to have a second set of stationery for marketing purposes you may want to include your e-mail and web site addresses as well as your fax number.

Stationery represents you and sometimes is how you make your first impression, just as business cards do. Give consideration to the font you choose, the boldness of the ink, and the colors of the paper and the ink. Yes, these do tell the public who you are. A very thin, less expensive paper stock gives the impression that you are unsuccessful or very cheap. In addition, paper that is too "classy" looking can seem ostentatious.

Colors are now commonly used by professional psychotherapists, rather than the traditional black ink on white paper. Even with color, however, be sure that you maintain a professional "look." Deep-color inks are usually more professional than are lighter pastels. However, you may choose a pastel stationery paper, especially if you specialize in infertility, breast cancer (the pink ribbon is the support symbol), or children. When choosing stationery, give thought to how consumers will think of you when they see what you use to represent yourself.

BUSINESS CARDS

Closely related to stationery, but more directly used for the purposes of promotion, are business cards. Psychotherapists typically use business cards as simple calling cards, as instruments that can be used to distribute their name, phone number, and address. Usually, the word or words "psychotherapist," "executive coach," "psychologist," "social worker," "sports psychologist," or "family counselor" and the appropriate degrees also appear. The exchange of business cards is a standard ritual for all professionals.

The same guidelines that are true for stationery hold for business cards. If your state requires your license number, it must appear. If you are incorporated, your corporation name must appear on the card. Consider choosing cards that match your stationery. The color of paper and ink and type of font look best when seen as a coordinated set.

Business cards are typically 2 inches by 3½ inches and are typeset at a printing shop or are desktop published on a high-quality specialty paper. The following list will give you a sense of some of the possibilities to consider.

Business card minimal essentials:

- name and degree
- address and phone number

- profession
- license number as required in some states

Business card options:

- distinctive color of print and/or card stock
- distinctive font and/or size
- one-sided, two-sided or specialty card
- e-mail and/or Web site address
- logo or artwork
- description of your services or professional background
- specialty location features such as free parking or well-known location (e.g., in a medical center or shopping complex)
- map or direction to office location
- branches of your office
- affiliations (e.g., professor at a particular university)
- recognizable honors (e.g., fellow of the American Psychological Association or Diplomate in National Association of Social Workers)
- names of associates and/or their specialties
- tag line: a descriptive sentence that tells people what makes you special and unique

Marketing with Business Cards

- Be sure to *always* have your business cards on hand.
- Use your business cards frequently—at social occasions, at business meetings, and during workshops or talks.
- In your office, use the back of your business cards as you would use notepaper to schedule patient's appointments or write referral information.
- Consider having two types of business cards: the simple generic inexpensive kind that you use as scrap paper and distribute continually and the more expensive marketing version that you distribute in networking settings and at business-related events.

A Marketing Example*

Karen Kalish, owner of a successful public relations firm and counsel to several large clients, including the APA, uses several types of business cards. At the end of media development workshops, she distributes a

---

* See the Appendix for information regarding materials described in this chapter.

six-part foldout card that summarizes the do's and don'ts of a successful press interview, including recommendations about appropriate manner of dress. This "business card" is wonderfully effective because of the pertinent advice. Karen follows her own public relations advice and her handout materials illustrate her effectiveness. After all, are you not more likely to find public relations experts more credible if their own materials are memorable?

Some Examples of Psychotherapists' Business Cards*

Sandra Haber

This card has a very traditional look (Figure 11.1). The font style and layout are traditional; however, the tag line at the very bottom is very new. It is an example of a foldover card that gives detailed information when opened.

Karyn Figlen Schorr and Leslie Davenport

In Figure 11.2, notice the practice name and its initials. This is a well-balanced card that is informative yet not overcrowded. Schorr and Davenport deal with separate locations by offering only a phone number.

Kate Hays

This card is presented vertically and this is its attraction (Figure 11.3). The card is filled with information yet does not look messy or too confusing. Use of different fonts and different sizes makes this work.

Gloria T. Paknis

Figure 11.4 is a card that reads almost like a curriculum vita. It lists Gloria's credentials as well as her specialty services. A card can give you much more space for information and messages.

---

* See the Appendix for information regarding materials described in this chapter.

Sandra Haber, Ph. D.

Licensed Psychologist
A fellow of the American Psychological Association

211 West 56 St., Suite 21 H
New York, New York 10019   Tel. (212) 246-6057

REDUCING THE TRAUMA OF CANCER FOR PATIENTS, PARTNERS AND FAMILIES

A

Dr. Sandra Haber, a fellow of the American Psychological
Association was honored as Distinguished Psychologist of the
Year in 1993-4 for her pioneering contributions in psycho-
oncology.

Dr. Haber edited *Breast Cancer: A Psychological Treatment
Manual* (Springer, 1995) and is co-author of *When Someone
You Love Has Prostate Cancer* (Delacourt).

Dr. Haber has a private practice in New York City.

USING THE MIND TO HEAL THE BODY . . .

- *Stress Interventions*
- *Imagery Training*
- *Self-Hypnosis*
- *Body Image and Sexual Adjustment*
- *Communication Skills*
- *Parenting and Family Concerns*

REDUCING THE TRAUMA OF CANCER FOR PATIENTS, PARTNERS AND FAMILIES

B

FIGURE 11.1   Sandra Haber's business card. **A:** Card when folded. **B:** Card
when unfolded.

Marketing Advisors for Professionals
New Directions For The Clinical Practitioner

• *Private Practice Training Workshops*
• *Marketing Focused Support Groups*
• *Individual Consultation*
• *Resource Library*

Karyn Figlen Schorr, C.S.W.
Leslie Davenport, C.S.W.   (212) 213-9768

FIGURE 11.2   Business card for Schorr and Davenport.

The
Performing
Edge

*Performance enhancement
training for the athlete,
performing artist,
and business person*

KATE F. HAYS, PH.D.
Psychologist
Certified Consultant, AAASP

52 Nassau Street
Toronto, ON   M5T 1M2

416.599-6528
FAX: 416.961-5516

Email:
The_Performing_Edge@compuserve.com

FIGURE 11.3   Business card for Kate Hays.

SOLUTIONS
For Stress

Where you'll find professional skill and compassionate care.

You have an appointment

on _____ at _____am pm

on _____ at _____am pm

on _____ at _____am pm

on _____ at _____am pm

on _____ at _____am pm

on _____ at _____am pm

If you are unable to keep your
appointment(s), please let us know
24 hours in advance.

REDUCE STRESS
- *Find relief from anxiety or panic*
- *Reduce organization absenteeism*
- *Individual and group counseling*
- *Stress management workshops*
- *Massage therapies*
- *Increase your overall health and vitality*

GLORIA T. PAKNIS, M.S.W., L.C.S.W.
Director
Education: M.S.W., New York University, Graduate School of Social Work
Advanced Work: The Metropolitan Institute for Training in
Psychoanalytic Psychotherapy
Board-Certified Diplomate
Member: NASW, MSPP, ACSW, SCSWP, NJAWT, MHAMC

37 Kings Road • Madison, NJ 07940
One block from Town Hall, across from the train station

973-377-3966 • *Fax* 973-377-5931

FIGURE 11.4   Business card for Gloria Paknis.

Chapter 12

Flyers, Newsletters, Fact Sheets, and Brochures

The next level of basic marketing tools typically involves an increase in both your time and your financial investment. Depending on the simplicity or grandeur of your style, you can expect flyers to be the fastest and most economical product and newsletter and brochures to be the most time consuming and expensive. However, for each product you choose to explore, there will still be a number of options, one of which will be right for your practice.

FLYERS

Flyers are the quick and easy way to market your practice. If you have access to a basic computer and printer or a copy machine, then you are in business. The basic flyer usually functions as an announcement. It tells people of an event that will take place. Most often, you will be using flyers to announce a talk, workshop or event you are hosting.

Flyer minimal essentials:

- your name, degree, and profession
- the title of workshop or talk
- the day, date, and time of the event
- the location of the event
- charges or fees
- phone number to call for more information (This is useful for individuals who want private appointments as well as for individuals who are interested but cannot attend on that particular date.)

Flyer options:

- information about your target audience (This workshop is for couples in second marriages.)
- bullet points that tell the reader what they will get from attending your talk (This talk will teach you three ways to reduce your stress.)
- any preregistration information or information about how and when to respond

Flyer production decisions:

- font styles and size of print
- color, weight, and size of paper. Note that flyers are cheap to produce, but you want the flyer to "fit" the event. A colored flyer might be appropriate for a singles event, but a beige flyer might be more appropriate for a talk on cancer. The standard 8½ inch by 11 inch sheet of paper is just that—standard. Consider asking for a different sized paper or one of a more substantial weight to make your flyer a bit different.
- logos, visuals, or photographs. These can be reprinted onto a flyer and can create a more personal touch. You can use a photo of yourself or of something that is related to your workshop or clip art from a standard book (available in most art and computer stores). Once you venture into these choices, the price may increase proportionately, so gage your financial investment here because it relates to the return on investment you are expecting.
- cut-off date for reservations if it is important to know how many attendees there will be
- directions to location of event

Flyer marketing "add-ons" to consider:

- discounts that will be available to attendees (All workshop participants will get 10% off on a book or future workshop.)
- giveaways, such as a list of resources, reprinted articles, tip sheets, and so on, on your stationery or with your business card attached
- consider providing "light refreshments"
- future announcements that list titles and dates of next few talks
- joint offerings that combine your talk with a panel of speakers (For example, a talk on infertility might be combined with a medical specialist and an adoption counselor. Also consider a joint production with a recognized group such as the YMCA or a local bookstore.)

- feature your talk in a desirable location, such as a coffee shop or bookstore or in a resort area or upscale mall
- mention special accommodations, such as wheelchair-accessible or child-friendly environment

Flyer distribution decisions

- Post on bulletin boards, and in community centers, shopping areas, synagogues and churches, preschool facilities, pediatricians' offices, preschool clubs, computer centers, health food stores, and so on. You can post anywhere there is a bulletin board.
- Stack in waiting rooms or on countertops if you are able to attend to them frequently to neaten the pile
- Fold into more permanent brochures that are distributed or enclosed in routine mailings to patients and colleagues
- Leave in your waiting room; reciprocate with other mental health professionals. Stacked flyers can often be left on countertops with magazines. These are typically found at local health clubs, physicians offices, parent-teacher association meetings, book club gatherings, and so on

Some Examples of Flyers

Example 1

Figure 12.1 shows an example of a spirited flyer for teens. Although there is considerable information here, the layout, the font size, and the use of a graphic make the flyer attractive and readable.

Example 2

Note the prominent sponsorship of the YM and YWHA and the words "Free Workshop" in Figure 12.2. This simple flyer gives the basic information in a clear and appealing manner. It is enhanced by the visual in the left hand corner. It was inexpensive to create and reproduce.

NEWSLETTERS

Newsletters are another marketing device that can keep your name out in front of the public. Printed newsletters can be as brief as two pages (4 sides) or as lengthy as a magazine. Newsletters have three major elements: content, production, and distribution.

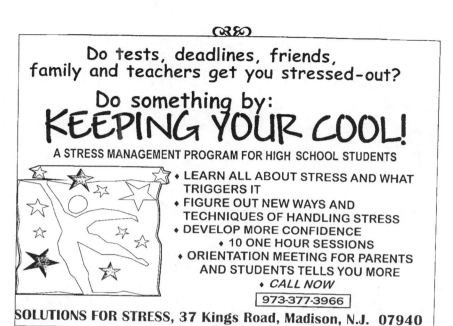

FIGURE 12.1 Example 1. Flyer for *Solutions for Stress.* (Used with permission of Gloria Paknis.)

The typical content of a newsletter might have a commentary from the editor, a feature article or main point, and an announcement section. It is the informational piece of the newsletter.

With desktop programs, the production of a brief newsletter can take place on your own computer. Some computers come already preloaded with such programs, or you can buy computer programs that will give you a preplanned layout in which you insert the text. Newsletter programs will typically have choices for font, layouts, and a variety of logos.

All newsletters need an outlet or manner of distribution. Who will get your newsletter, and how will they receive it? Will it be left in shops, professional offices, or your waiting room or will it be sent to a mailing list? One entrepreneurial individual we know leaves her newsletters in a basket outside her office building.[1] Passersby have learned to look for them and find the psychology education interesting and valuable, and her name recognition has been increased in the community at large.

PARENTING CENTER OF THE CENTRAL QUEENS YM&YWHA PRESENTS A FREE WORKSHP "OVERCOMING THE CHALLENGES OF INFERTILITY"

WITH DR. JANET MUELLER, PSY.D.

LICENSED PSYCHOLOGIST

SUNDAY, APRIL 5TH, 1998

10:00 TO 11:00 AM

PLEASE PRE-REGISTER WITH HOPE

268-5011 EXT. 240 OR STOP IN

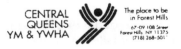

CENTRAL
QUEENS
YM & YWHA

The place to be
in Forest Hills

67-09 108 Street
Forest Hills, NY 11375
(718) 268-5011

FIGURE 12.2 Example 2. Flyer for *Overcoming the Challenges of Infertility*. (Used with permission of Janet Mueller and the Central Queens YM & YWHA.)

Considerations in Developing a Newsletter

There are numerous issues to consider if you are developing a newsletter. It takes a fair amount of time to write a newsletter or to recruit content materials and to set up and graphically lay out for desktop publishing. How often will your newsletter appear? Will it appear weekly, monthly, bimonthly, semi-annually, or annually? Can you keep up with the deadlines for production? Do you have enough content for an ongoing newsletter? Second, paper newsletters can become costly, especially if you need professional help with production. You should also factor in the costs of distribution, particularly if you are anticipating mailing the newsletter. For some newsletters with large or specialized distributions, outside advertising fees provide a cost offset, if you are willing and able to recruit the advertisers.

Enterprising individuals may also want to consider an online newsletter (in addition to or instead of the paper version). These newsletters (called e-zines) are circulated online through their Internet Web site, which significantly lowers the cost of production and distribution and increases the size of your potential audience. The specifics are presented in chapter 17 about Web sites and e-zines.

FACT SHEETS

Fact sheets can be an effective marketing tool. You can have a series of fact sheets on a variety of topics that you can use when marketing for that particular niche. The fact sheet is just that: facts of interest and importance for individuals to know about a particular topic. For example, if you are preparing a talk on work stress for your chamber of commerce, you may want to develop a fact sheet on signs of stress and tips on stress management.

The fact sheet can be created under your usual letterhead, or you can create a new letterhead for this purpose. Include your name, address, phone and fax, e-mail and Web site addresses if you choose.

Fact sheets can be printed from your own computer, allowing you to play with a variety of colors and fonts. If you are planning to have them reproduced, then standard black ink is the least expensive choice on plain, or color paper or on paper with a ready-made design, depending on what suits your topic and budget.

Fact sheets can be narrative or bulleted style. Your professional organization may have a fact sheet on a number of topics. The following example is a fact sheet produced by the APA on anxiety disorders (Figure 12.3). Although it is loaded with information, note that it is also written in a reader-friendly and narrative style. To personalize this fact sheet, you might consider stapling your business card on the top left side.

Sometimes, your professional association does not have a fact sheet related to the topic you are interested in, or the materials on the fact sheet or article do not quite fit your needs. In this case, you can simply develop your own bulleted fact sheet that gives the information you consider to be important. Sources for this information can be books, articles, or other professionally reliable materials. These sources should be cited at the end of the fact sheet.

Figure 12.4 is an example of a briefer bulleted fact sheet excerpted from Figure 12.3.

BROCHURES

Brochures are a wonderful method of giving out information about your professional niche or service. Brochures can be designed simply and inexpensively, and desktop programs are readily available.

An attractive brochure can lend a professional and polished image to your business and is an attractive summary of the services you offer. However, compared with business cards, flyers, and fact sheets, brochures are far more time consuming to develop and are expensive to produce.

The following suggestions apply to the typical trifold, six-paneled brochure. Follow along with the description provided by making a mock brochure for yourself. Take a sheet of paper and fold it into thirds as you would a letter going into an envelope. Open the paper and hold it horizontally. Number the inside panels (the page facing you) 1, 2, and 3 from left to right. Turn the sheet over and number the panels again from left to right 4, 5, and 6. Refold the paper into thirds. Now follow along.

Designing Your Brochure

The cover of the brochure (the one third of the page that is facing you) is actually panel 6. Its attractiveness is critical to the success of your brochure. The cover should have the subject of your brochure presented in an appealing manner. It should draw the readers in and make them want to open the brochure, read your message, and save it. Often, this can be accomplished through an interesting graphic, question, or tag line. Although this brochure panel typically has the fewest words, it needs to be the most intriguing. How the cover looks will determine whether the brochure will be opened or overlooked.

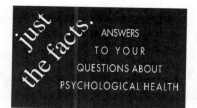

Anxiety Disorders:
The Role of Psychotherapy in Effective Treatment

Everyone feels anxious and under stress from time to time. Situations such as meeting tight deadlines, important social obligations or driving in heavy traffic, often bring about anxious feelings. Such mild anxiety may help make you alert and focused on facing threatening or challenging circumstances. On the other hand, anxiety disorders cause severe distress over a period of time and disrupt the lives of individuals suffering from them. The frequency and intensity of anxiety involved in these disorders is often debilitating. But fortunately, with proper and effective treatment, people suffering from anxiety disorders can lead normal lives.

. . . .

What are the major kinds of anxiety disorders?

There are several major types of anxiety disorders, each with its own characteristics.

❖ People with **generalized anxiety disorder** have recurring fears or worries, such as about health or finances, and they often have a persistent sense that something bad is just about to happen. The reason for the intense feelings of anxiety may be difficult to identify. But the fears and worries are very real and often keep individuals from concentrating on daily tasks.

❖ **Panic disorder** involves sudden, intense and unprovoked feelings of terror and dread. People who suffer from this disorder generally develop strong fears about when and where their next panic attack will occur, and they often restrict their activities as a result.

❖ A related disorder involves **phobias**, or intense fears, about certain objects or situations. Specific phobias may involve things such as encountering certain animals or flying in airplanes, whereas social phobias involve fear of social settings or public places.

❖ **Obsessive-compulsive disorder** is characterized by persistent, uncontrollable and unwanted feelings or thoughts (obsessions) and routines or rituals in which individuals engage to try to prevent or rid themselves

of these thoughts (compulsions). Examples of common compulsions include washing hands or cleaning house excessively for fear of germs, or checking over something repeatedly for errors.

❖ Someone who suffers severe physical or emotional trauma such as from a natural disaster or serious accident or crime may experience **post-traumatic stress disorder**. Thoughts, feelings and behavior patterns become seriously affected by reminders of the event, sometimes months or even years after the traumatic experience.

Symptoms such as shortness of breath, racing heartbeat, trembling and dizziness often accompany certain anxiety disorders such as panic and generalized anxiety disorders. Although they may begin at any time, anxiety disorders often surface in adolescence or early adulthood. There is some evidence of a genetic or family predisposition to certain anxiety disorders.

Why is it important to seek treatment for these disorders?

If left untreated, anxiety disorders can have severe consequences. For example, some people who suffer from recurring panic attacks avoid at all costs putting themselves in a situation that they fear may trigger an attack. Such avoidance behavior may create problems by conflicting with job requirements, family obligations or other basic activities of daily living.

FIGURE 12.3 Example 3: APA anxiety disorder fact sheet. (Used with permission of the American Psychological Association.)

Many people who suffer from an untreated anxiety disorder are prone to other psychological disorders, such as depression, and they have a greater tendency to abuse alcohol and other drugs. Their relationships with family members, friends and coworkers may become very strained. And their job performance may falter.

Are there effective treatments available for anxiety disorders?

Absolutely. Most cases of anxiety disorder can be treated successfully by appropriately trained health and mental health care professionals.

According to the National Institute of Mental Health, research has demonstrated that both "behavioral therapy" and "cognitive therapy" can be highly effective in treating anxiety disorders. Behavioral therapy involves using techniques to reduce or stop the undesired behavior associated with these disorders. For example, one approach involves training patients in relaxation and deep breathing techniques to counteract the agitation and hyperventilation (rapid, shallow breathing) that accompany certain anxiety disorders.

Through cognitive therapy, patients learn to understand how their thoughts contribute to the symptoms of anxiety disorders, and how to change those thought patterns to reduce the likelihood of occurrence and the intensity of reaction. The patient's increased cognitive awareness is often combined with behavioral techniques to help the individual gradually confront and tolerate fearful situations in a controlled, safe environment.

Proper and effective medications may have a role in treatment along with psychotherapy. In cases where medications are used, the patient's care may be managed collaboratively by a therapist and physician. It is important for patients to realize that there are side effects to any drugs, which must be monitored closely by the prescribing physician.

How can a qualified therapist help someone suffering from an anxiety disorder?

Licensed psychologists are highly qualified to diagnose and treat anxiety disorders. Individuals suffering from these disorders should seek a provider who is competent in cognitive and behavioral therapies. Experienced mental health professionals have the added benefit of having helped other patients recover from anxiety disorders.

Family psychotherapy and group psychotherapy (typically involving individuals who are not related to one another) offer helpful approaches to treatment for some patients with anxiety disorders. In addition, mental health clinics or other specialized treatment programs dealing with specific disorders such as panic or phobias may also be available nearby.

How long does psychological treatment take?

It is very important to understand that treatments for anxiety disorders do not work instantly. The patient should be comfortable from the outset with the general treatment being proposed and with the therapist with whom he or she is working. The patient's cooperation is crucial, and there must be a strong sense that the patient and therapist are collaborating as a team to remedy the anxiety disorder.

No one plan works well for all patients. Treatment needs to be tailored to the needs of the patient and to the type of disorder, or disorders, from which the individual suffers. A therapist and patient should work together to assess whether a treatment plan seems to be on track. Adjustments to the plan sometimes are necessary, since patients respond differently to treatment.

Many patients will begin to improve noticeably within eight to ten sessions, especially those who carefully follow the outlined treatment plan.

There is no question that the various kinds of anxiety disorders can severely impair a person's functioning in work, family and social environments. But the prospects for long-term recovery for most individuals who seek appropriate professional help are very good. Those who suffer from anxiety disorders can work with a qualified and experienced therapist such as a licensed psychologist to help them regain control of their feelings and thoughts -- and their lives.

October 1998
This document may be reproduced in its entirety with no modifications.

AMERICAN
PSYCHOLOGICAL
ASSOCIATION

Talk to Someone Who Can Help
800-964-2000

750 First Street NE
Washington, DC 20002-4242

FIGURE 12.3 Example 3: APA anxiety disorder fact sheet (*continued*).

[Your Letterhead]

A FACT SHEET ON ANXIETY DISORDERS

People with anxiety disorders usually have recurring fears or worries. They spend a great deal of their time with a sense that something bad is about to happen. There are several different types of anxiety disorders, each with a slightly different set of symptoms and each with a different name. For example, sometimes there is a stronger, more intense feeling of terror or dread that we call a "panic attack." When it happens, the person will often spend time worrying about when and where the next panic attack will occur. Another type of anxiety disorder is called a phobia, which is characterized by a very intense, specific fear about a certain object or situation. Sometimes, the anxiety disorder appears as a series of persistent, uncontrollable thoughts or behaviors. This is called obsessive-compulsive disorder. Lastly, some anxiety disorders are a result of a specific physical or emotional traumatic event, such as a rape, plane crash, or crime. This is called post-traumatic stress disorder.

- It's important to treat an anxiety disorder for the following reasons:
  - The person may begin to avoid many situations because he or she is afraid of feeling anxious. This can create problems with job requirements, family living, and other basic activities.
  - untreated anxiety disorders can lead to other problems such as depression, alcohol or drug abuse, and stressful and strained relationships.
  - anxiety disorders interfere with the quality of people's lives, causing them to limit and restrict their activities out of worry and fear.
- Anxiety disorders CAN BE HELPED
  - Behavioral therapy can teach patients to relax and counteract the agitation and physical responses to an anxiety disorder.
  - Cognitive therapy helps patients learn to change their thought patterns, thereby reducing the likelihood and intensity of anxiety reactions.
  - Proper medications may be suggested to manage symptoms while the person is learning new anxiety management techniques.

A licensed psychotherapist is qualified to diagnose and treat anxiety disorders. Feel free to contact "Your name" for more information.

FIGURE 12.4 Example 4. A bulleted fact sheet on anxiety disorders. (Modified, with permission, from APA: *Anxiety disorders: The role of psychotherapy in effective treatment*. See Figure 12.3).

Clip art, available in books at art stores and on computer disks is an inexpensive way to have access to graphics. Some photographs can also be successfully printed on a brochure and graphic artists have a wide range of prices. If you are on a budget, consider hiring a student at a school for graphic arts. If you are willing to shop around, you may well be able to find a graphic artist within your budget.

In Figure 12.5 note the dramatic difference in appeal of two straight-talk brochures. Both were designed by professional graphic artists, but the first (Fig. 12.5A) uses type changes to create interest, the second (Fig. 12.5B) uses a photograph and an intriguing message. Which brochure would catch your interest?

Panels 1, 2, 3 are the three inside panels of the brochure when it is completely opened. These panels typically state the topic, the problem, and exactly how you are going to help the reader. This is the text of your brochure, and it is time consuming to write.

We recommend the use of bullets, type changes, and succinct statements to get your message across. Remember, no psychobabble! These are the panels that will sell your work. They need to give the readers a sense that you know your specialty and have clear and definite solutions to their problem.

Panels 4 and 5 are the left and middle panels when the brochure is open and turned over. Depending on your material, these panels may have more text, a list of other services provided, biographical information about you, your photo, and additional graphics.

Typically, panel 5 (center back) has more white space than the other panels. Here you can print your name, office address, logo, telephone number and Web site. If the brochure is to be a self-mailer (stapled or taped shut), and not put into an envelop, then this panel might simply have your return address at the top. The rest of the panel would be saved for the address of the recipient and the postage.

Rick Weiss,[2] owner of Desktop Media of Phoenix, Arizona, suggests avoiding too much content. "This is a promotional piece, not a statement of all of your views." Other issues to keep in mind when writing text are as follows:

- Make sure that the important issues are clearly marked.
- Keep the design style consistent throughout.
- Use type faces that are clean (easy on the eyes). Do not use more than two or three fonts.

Brochure Production Decisions

- Use quality stock paper. The weight of the paper should be substantial (at least 80 lb). Do not cut corners. You do not want to print a brochure on flimsy paper.

"I knew that I could talk

about anything and

Straight Talk:

everything with my

Choosing

psychologist — and that

a Psychologist

I would not be judged.

Our conversations not only

gave me the acceptance

I needed, but practical

wisdom as well."

A

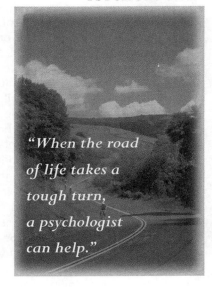

CHOOSING A
PSYCHOLOGIST

*"When the road
of life takes a
tough turn,
a psychologist
can help."*

B

FIGURE 12.5A, B: Example 5—Straight talk brochures.

- Artwork. A clear photo or drawing can be used successfully. Stock art can be obtained at a range of prices (sometimes quite affordable) from stock photo houses. Also consider clip art and other computer-generated graphics.
- Color. One-color ink is less expensive than is two-color; two-color processing is less expensive than three-color processing, and so on. Remember that a one-color process also includes varying shades of a color, and interesting effects can be achieved. Do not mix bright and bold colors with soft or pastel colors. If you are going to use bright, keep all the colors bright. If soft, stay soft.
- If you are technologically able, or at least technologically willing, consider producing your own brochures on your desktop. The results can be professional, the text can be changed at will, and the costs are a fraction of professional production. Programs such as Printmaster® offer easy-to-use templates.
- If you work with a graphic designer, the fee is usually "per job" rather than per hour to give the designer flexibility in how much time his or her "creativity" takes. Get an estimate of the overall package (job fee) so that if the designer takes longer than estimated, it is at their expense. The time it takes for the designer to do a brochure depends on how much you provide the designer. A typical brochure can be set up easily in 1 or 2 hours. Costs are also affected by whether there are photographs to input, logos to be designed or specific kinds of art to be used. Most designers will charge additional fees if you make changes after the original work is completed, so you must clarify this issue ahead of time. Corrections (mistakes by the designer), however, are a part of the original quote (or should be). Also note that many designers are good at copy writing. They will charge extra, but they will have a good sense of what works.
- Holding costs down. The most expensive element in brochure production can be printing the job if there has not been proofing. It is the reruns that kill you financially. Proof, proof, and proof again. Then have someone else proof it! Have a friend who is unfamiliar with the information proof it; this person will be less likely to skim over some routine words.
- Color is a key issue when considering cost. If you are on a tight budget, use paper that has the colors in it, and then stick with a one-color ink, usually black.
- Quantity is related to costs, and the rule of thumb is that prices get considerably cheaper the more you print, but why print more than you will ever use? Be mindful of how timely the information is. Are you sending it out in large mailings up front, in small

amounts as they are requested, or just leaving them around for people to pick up? The slower the distribution, the smaller the quantity you want.

Some Examples of Brochure

Example 1

This brochure (Figure 12.6) captivates the reader through the use of a fluid graphic that ties in with the topic of performance. The inside text offers a clear explanation of the services offered. This brochure also offers a personal message from Kate Hays, sports psychologist, as well as an appealing photo. Note that the rear panel is blank and can serve as a place for mailing labels.

Example 2

Figure 12.7 uses both simple drawings and a variety of type styles and bold lettering to achieve visual ease for the reader.

Example 3

This brochure (Figure 12.8) is attractive because it immediately asks the reader questions about his or her needs. It gives considerable information about the author and several short testimonials about her work. Notice that the brochure is in lowercase letters and uses only two fonts with some bold highlights for emphasis.

Example 4

A four-sided brochure with open space that is appealing is seen in Figure 12.9. They use a triangular logo on the outside and carry it over to the inside in the same color, which makes your eye follow the design. Clear short statements about the purpose give the reader ideas to consider.

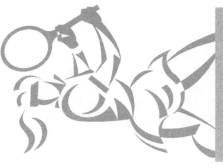

Performance enhancement training is an individually designed and systematic way to improve your performance through the use of specific mental skills.

IT IS DESIGNED TO:

• Overcome performance blocks through positive thinking, attention and focused concentration.

• Develop individualized performance goals that are challenging, realistic and measurable.

• Find your optimal level of performance tension.

• Increase your confidence in your performance through understanding the relationship between your mind and your body in demanding and high stress situations.

• Help you achieve peak performance through mental rehearsal and visualization training.

PERFORMANCE ENHANCEMENT TRAINING IS AVAILABLE IN THE FOLLOWING WAYS:

• **Individual, hourly sessions** focus on specific problem areas and their resolution, and suggest new methods for enhancing your performance.

• **Small Group sessions** (3-5 hours over a 2-3 week period) provide individuals with group support and recognition of problems and performance issues. This approach is especially useful for existing teams or groups. It can also be adapted to athletes or businesses with shared interests.

• **Workshops** are designed to introduce participants to basic performance enhancement concepts with special focus on tension management, imagery training and self-talk. Both introductory and day long workshops are available.

• **Consultation** can benefit coaches, athletic directors, physical educators, and business persons who want to help others achieve optimal performance.

• **Case Consultation** is also useful for physicians and physical therapists, coaches, personal trainers and others working with individual athletes. Consultation is available on a one-time or on-going basis.

• **Supervision** is designed for psychologists, other mental health professionals and educators developing expertise in sport and performance psychology.

I get such enjoyment out of helping people become their best. While formal preparation is vital, it often doesn't address the mental aspects of performance. Sweaty palms, mentally beating yourself up if your performance isn't perfect, having trouble staying focused—these are all common mental responses to performance expectations. Performance enhancement training assists people in developing the skills to handle their minds so their bodies can perform optimally. People incorporate many ideas and mental skills within a few sessions. They feel more confident in their own capacities.

—Kate Hays

FIGURE 12.6A   Example 1: Brochure for *The Performing Edge*, panels 1–3.

The
Performing
Edge

Performance enhancement training for the athlete, performing artist and business person

KATE F. HAYS, PH.D., C.PSYCH.

730 Yonge Street Suite 226
Toronto, ON M4Y 2B7
(416) 961-0487 Fax: (416) 961-5516
The_Performing_Edge@compuserve.com

Sport Psychology Consultant
Toronto Sports & Exercise Medicine Institute (SEMI)
4779 Yonge Street
Toronto, ON M2N 5M5
(416) 223-SEMI

**The
Performing
Edge**

KATE F. HAYS, PHD, CPSYCH
Practise in Clinical/Sport Psychology
Certified Consultant, AAASP

KATE F. HAYS, PH.D, C.PSYCH., established a practise in clinical and sport/performance psychology in Toronto in 1998, after a 25 year career in psychology in the U.S. Her focus on performance enhancement includes work with individuals, small groups, and large group workshops. She brings additional personal energy and creativity to this work through her own involvement as a runner and musician.

Dr. Hays has lectured widely throughout North America. Her combined interests in exercise and psychotherapy have resulted in two recent books, *Working It Out: Using Exercise in Therapy* (APA, 1999) and the edited *Integrating Exercise, Sports, Movement, and Mind: Therapeutic Unity* (Haworth, 1998). She is a Fellow of the American Psychological Association; a Certified Consultant, Association for the Advancement of Applied Sport Psychology; and listed in the United States Olympic Committee Sport Psychology Registry. She has held a number of elected positions within the APA's Division of Exercise and Sport Psychology.

FIGURE 12.6B   Example 1: Brochure for *The Performing Edge*, panels 4–6. (Used with permission of Kate Hays.)

Did You Know...?

Stress on the job led 34% of all American employees to consider quitting their jobs.[1]

Stress can cause decreased productivity, absenteeism, illness, employee turnover, even theft and sabotage costing American employers an estimated $1,700 per employee annually.[2]

20% of Americans surveyed in a recent poll said that stress had interfered with their ability to do their job.[3]

IS THIS HAPPENING AT YOUR COMPANY!

WHAT CAN BE DONE?

WHO HAS THE SOLUTIONS?

1 Northwestern National Life Insurance Company
2 "About Half Suffer From Stress Due to Job, Gallup Poll Says," Desert News, January 11, 1990
3 "About Half Suffer

Let SOLUTIONS FOR STRESS be your guide to gaining control of your stress...

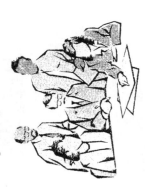

Mobile Programs accommodate busy schedules

Our Mobile Programs, consisting of training, presentations, and on-site massage, accommodate busy schedules by bringing the solutions to your workplace.

These customized programs are for individuals, corporations, businesses, professional associations, municipalities, law enforcement agencies and more. They teach the essential concepts, strategies, and techniques of stress management.

On-site Corporate Programs decrease workplace stress and increase productivity

Our On-site Corporate Programs are individually tailored and designed to create beneficial scenarios for both the employer and the 46% of American employees who find their job stressful.[4]

Employees learn to identify, reduce and manage their stress while employers experience decreased absenteeism and increased levels of productivity.

Our programs consist of options ranging from individual to departmental consultations to our corporate specific training workshops such as "Controlling Workplace Stress" and "Time Management."

Professional Massage reduces stress and relieves tension related headaches and eye strain.

The release of muscular tension helps to unblock and balance the overall flow of life energy throughout the body. On-site seated or table massage can be provided at your office.

4 "Stress in Workplace is Rising, Survey Says," Desert News, May 8: 1991, 3A.

FIGURE 12.7A   Example 2: Brochure for *Solutions for Stress*, panels 1–3.

STRESS...

It's A
Fact
of Life.
But Can
You Live
With It?

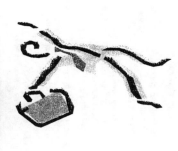

SOLUTIONS
For Stress.

Where you'll find professional skill and compassionate care.

Director and Founder

Gloria T. Paknis, MSW, LCSW, Director and Founder of SOLUTIONS FOR STRESS, is a 20 year veteran in the field of Stress Management. She is an expert in the proven techniques of successful stress management:

Self-Monitoring

Cognitive Restructuring

Environmental Engineering

Formal Relaxation Training

Based on her expertise and under her direction, SOLUTIONS FOR STRESS provides specially designed stress management programs for individuals, businesses, organizations, and corporations.

Let SOLUTIONS FOR STRESS be your guide to gaining control of your stress.

Our licensed and certified professionals are experts in all aspects of stress management.

For Complete Details

SOLUTIONS
For Stress.

37 Kings Road
Madison, NJ 07940

973-377-3966

Fax: 973-377-5931

50% of all Americans say that job stress affects their health, relationships and job performance.[5]

A Sampling of Program Topics

Workplace Stress

Time Management

Assertiveness Training

Managing Your Anger

Trouble Shooting Corporate Transitions

Living with Stress & Staying Healthy

Relaxation Training

Spatial Restructuring

Self-Massage

Stress Induced Eating

Family Stress

Creative Visualization

Teens; Keeping Your Cool!

5 "Stress in Workplace is Rising, Survey Says," Desert News, May 8: 1991, 3A.

FIGURE 12.7B Example 2: Brochure for *Solutions for Stress*, panels 4–6. (Used with permission of Gloria T. Paknis, Solutions for Stress.)

why has rosemary had such success helping clients find work they love?

rosemary lavinski, M.S.W., B.C.D., is a seasoned social worker and career management consultant who is down-to-earth, practical and aware of market trends. When you are ready to make the moves that allow for growth and change she can:

§ help you analyze your interests, clarify your values and recognize what gives you pleasure so you can find the work you love

§ assist you in managing office politics so you can play to win

§ coach you to be a good team player in your present job so you become an indispensable asset to your organization

§ teach you how to package your skills strategically so you can target your market

§ show you how to tap into the hidden job market and improve your networking techniques

§ collaborate with you to create resumes and cover letters that are attention getting and based on your strengths, abilities and goals

§ point out how to identify personality types and communication styles of potential employers to give you an edge in interviews

§ interpret your personality and interest inventory testing with an understanding of the power of unconscious habits and longings so you can make changes

what makes rosemary unique?

She is a solution-oriented social work psychotherapist which enhances her expertise in career management. Able to uncover the causes that keep you stuck, in work or in life, her guidance and support assist you to mobilize your resources, feel more connected and more alive. She helps you:

§ manage your personal, marital, family and work stresses more effectively

§ balance sharing, intimacy and love with individuality and assertiveness

§ work at your own pace

rosemary works in groups of eight or less and, of course, one on one. Results are apparent in six sessions of career counseling. Even faster, if individual sessions can be scheduled.

Why stay stuck when there is a way out? Accept that you can take charge and make changes.

rosemary lavinski, M.S.W., B.C.D. has helped people in
business and finance
the legal profession
the creative and helping professions
move on to rewarding
love lives
work lives
family relationships

"rosemary is chock full of practical information. I got much more than I expected." A financial analyst

"rosemary saved my life. I no longer am depressed and am more spiritually aware. I never knew I could feel so good." A social worker

"rosemary interpreted my personality testing in a way that showed me where my strengths are and helped me develop a plan to meet my personal and professional goals." A lawyer

career transition groups
manhattan:
wednesday 7:15 - 8:45PM
brooklyn:
thursday 7:30 - 9:00PM
psychotherapy group
manhattan:
monday 7:00 - 8:30PM
by appointment
718-783-4295 or 212-473-6836

Fees may be insurance reimbursable

FIGURE 12.8A   Example 3: Brochure from Rosemary Lavinski, panels 1–3.

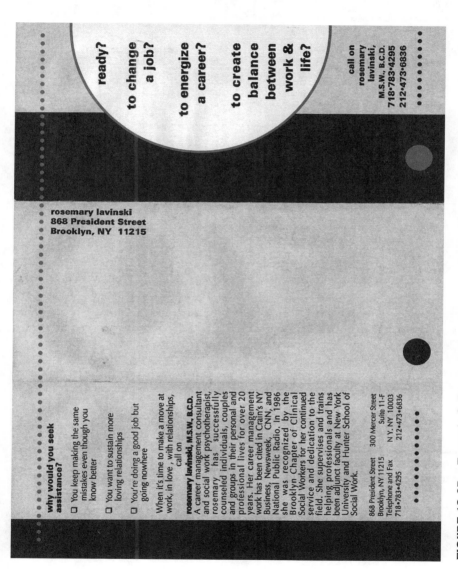

why would you seek assistance?

☐ You keep making the same mistakes even though you know better

☐ You want to sustain more loving relationships

☐ You're doing a good job but going nowhere

When it's time to make a move at work, in love , with relationships, call on

rosemary lavinski, M.S.W., B.C.D.
A career management consultant and social work psychotherapist, rosemary has successfully counseled individuals, couples and groups in their personal and professional lives for over 20 years. Her career management work has been cited in Crain's NY Business, Newsweek, CNN, and National Public Radio. In 1986 she was recognized by the Brooklyn Chapter of Clinical Social Workers for her continued service and dedication to the field. She supervises and trains helping professionals and has been adjunct faculty at New York University and Hunter School of Social Work.

868 President Street
Brooklyn, NY 11215
Telephone and Fax
718•783•4295

300 Mercer Street
Suite 11-F
N.Y, NY 10003
212•473•6836

rosemary lavinski
868 President Street
Brooklyn, NY 11215

ready?

to change a job?

to energize a career?

to create balance between work & life?

call on
rosemary
lavinski,
M.S.W., B.C.D.
718•783•4295
212•473•6836

FIGURE 12.8B Example 3: Brochure from Rosemary Lavinski, panels 4–6. (Used with permission of Rosemary Lavinski.)

You are in the Middle Years of Your Life!

Mid-Life Mentors Can Help You

Are You Wondering Whether the Next Years of Your Life Will Be Years of Loss and Decline?

You have been bombarded with negative images of what it means to be "middle aged." Can you still feel good about yourself? Can you still feel like an attractive and vital person?

No Question About It!

You might be surprised to hear what recent studies have shown:

Despite the stresses and challenges of the middle years, many men and women experience middle age as an exciting and deeply rewarding time of life.

So What is the Key to a Sense of Psychological Well Being in Mid-Life?

> *New Learning*
> *New Growth*
> *New Self-Discovery*

In Our Workshops, Lectures and Support Groups You Will Learn to:

▶ Discard the negative images of mid-life as a time of decline

▶ Discover the opportunity for personal growth and fulfillment inherent in the middle years

▶ Develop untapped resources in yourself

▶ Capitalize on your experience, knowledge and accomplishments as you frame new goals

▶ Challenge self-imposed limitations on your professional and financial success

▶ Recharge your spirit of curiosity and adventure

▶ Understand the most important differences between men and women in mid-life

Mid-Life Mentors

FIGURE 12.9A   Example 4: Brochure from Mid-Life Mentors, panels 1–3.

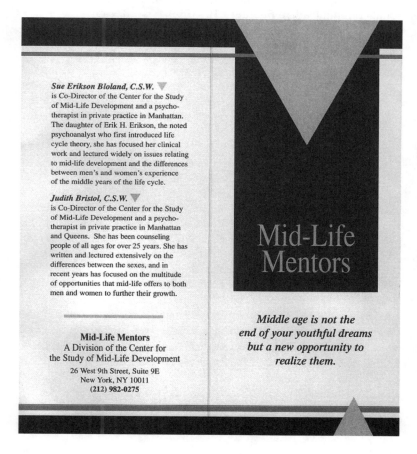

FIGURE 12.9B Example 4: Brochure from Mid-Life Mentors, panels 4–6. (Used with permission of Mid-Life Mentors, a division of the Center for the Study of Mid-Life Development.)

NOTES

[1] M. Jaffe, personal communication, April 10, 1999.
[2] Personal communication, February 10, 1999.

Part V

Intermediate Tools of the Trade

Chapter 13

Speeches and Workshops

SPEECHES

The anxiety connected to public speaking is considered to be one of the most prevalent worries. Although most psychotherapists have managed to get through a required undergraduate class in speechmaking, few have the skills or confidence to use this experience as the foundation for their a professional marketing.

Excellence in public speaking involves the mastery of two factors: content and performance. With some investment of time and practice, both of these factors can be shaped and polished to create a powerful and effective showcase for your skills as a psychotherapist.

If you choose to use speechmaking as part of your marketing strategy, it will help to have a thorough understanding of the ingredients it takes to be a memorable speaker.

Content of a Speech

A speech can be relatively brief. Even if you are allotted 40 minutes, you may decide to deliver a 20-minute talk and then spend the remaining 20 minutes fielding questions from the audience. Some people prefer this format because it appears informal, and they are more certain that they will be fulfilling the needs of the audience. Others prefer to fully prepare their talk for the total amount of time allotted. This choice will suit those of you who feel that you are the expert and the audience has come to hear your information. It also works well for attendees who may not be interested in your answers to other people's questions.

Again, the choice often depends on both your personal style and the topic and forum for the talk.

If you have a specialty and if you have achieved a gold standard of training and experience in a specific area, gathering your information for a talk should be quite easy. If you are a generalist, think of the kinds of issues you usually encounter with your patients. Focus on trying to identify specific issues that would be suitable for a talk. Do your research at the library or on the Internet and write your talk. Realize that whether you are the specialist or generalist, you have information that is worthwhile for others. They will appreciate your information and will think of you when they want help with this specific issue or other emotional difficulties.

Giving a good talk takes planning and preparation. You need to know not only your subject matter but also to whom you are speaking and what you want them to know. In *The Power of Public Speaking,* Marie Stuttgard (1997) suggests that before you accept an invitation to speak at any conference, inquire about the organization and what they will want from you. "Ask who they are, what they do, why they want you, and how they found you." It is this information that will help you make a decision about whether to accept the invitation. If you agree to speak, it will help you design your talk to fit in with the overall program, other speakers, and the audience. Think preparation, practice and presentation.

Karen Kalish suggests 10 steps for speech preparation:

1. Analyze your target audience.
2. Define what you want to communicate.
3. Research the issues.
4. Write a one-sentence objective in 25 words or less.
5. List three points you want to make.
6. Give an example, story, or anecdote to illustrate each point.
7. Write the opening of the speech.
8. Write the close of the speech.
9. Write the entire speech, making transitions from one section to another.
10. Prepare visual aids, if you are using them.

(Tip Sheet available: see Appendix)

Key Advice on Content

Karen Kalish suggests that you always remember that the audience is always asking WIIFM—What's In It For Me? Of course she suggests NBB—Never Be Boring.

Performance of a Speech

For most, public speaking requires a great deal of rehearsal. Very successful speakers appear natural at the podium but typically put in many hours of behind-the-scene preparation and rehearsal. Rehearsal is necessary for you to become familiar with the thoughts you want to communicate. By saying your talk aloud, you can hear it as the audience will hear it. You may want to tape yourself and play it back. For some, writing a very thorough outline is better than writing out the speech, mainly because you do not want to look stiff while standing and reading a speech. Think about having a conversation with the audience. You are probably quite capable of talking about your topic with one other person. Talking to 25 people is basically the same. Each individual is there to learn from what you have to say—talk to each individual.

Marie McDermott,[1] social worker–psychotherapist, discussed how difficult it was for her to speak publicly. When she was first asked, she would bring written notes, with comments about when to breathe, pause, and so on. As she became more proficient, she began to enjoy speaking and now finds that after a presentation people call her to ask about becoming a patient, make a referral, or ask her about supervision. Clearly, she has developed a relaxed, engaging style attractive to her audience.

Rehearsal is also necessary to gauge your length of speaking time. If you are on a panel, you may only have 10 minutes. If you are giving a talk at a parents meeting you may need to fill an hour. The best way to be sure that your estimate is accurate is to say the speech aloud and time yourself. This is especially important so you can make all your important points before you are stopped in your tracks by a panel chairperson. Rushing at the end of your talk confuses the audience, increases your anxiety, and often causes you to omit pertinent information.

If you are still anxious about public speaking but want to master it look into attending Toastmasters. Toastmasters, a nonprofit organization with low dues, will advise you on your speaking and communication skills in addition to giving you a place to practice and get feedback on your speech (1-800 WE SPEAK and http://www.toastmasters.org). Many active speakers mention that they have used Toastmaster programs and have reported that this experience helped them to break the ice of making speeches.

If all else fails and the adrenaline rush freezes you instead of energizing you, speak to your physician about using a beta-blocker medication to reduce your anxiety symptoms to slow your heart rate and lower your blood pressure during public speaking. Performers who need to have a steady hand and a clear mind are often prescribed this medication to be taken on an as needed basis. Persons who shake, sweat uncontrollably, and have a trembling voice or other phobic symptoms typically find this medication helpful.

Key Advice on Performance

Karen Kalish (How to give a terrific presentation, 1999) advises her clients to expect and accept nervousness. "You need to know that it's that adrenaline rush that will help you do a better job. So don't fight it." She also suggests that to manage excess stage fright you can walk up and down stairs, do isometric exercise, take deep breaths, or meditate, or a combination of these. (Karen Kalish Media Kit, see Appendix for contact information.)

WORKSHOPS

Workshops typically focus on achieving more goals than speeches do. One of these goals is usually to impart knowledge to the attendees, resulting in increased competence in the topic. You, the workshop leader, are the designated expert, and the participants are there to learn specific information or skills, or both, from you. For this reason it is usually a good idea to get feedback about your effectiveness as a workshop leader. A workshop evaluation completed by the attendees will give you a sense of how effective you were in communicating your information and whether you met the participant's expectations.

Ideas for Workshops

A novel idea for a workshop comes from Arthur Kovacs.[2]

> I am about to undertake a new venture. One of my best friends is an accountant. He has lost two huge financial management accounts and is now scared about his future. I told him we were going to design a workshop we will do together on coping with separation and divorce. I will take care of emotional and psychological needs; he can advise about finances and tax implications. We will get lots of new cases from these workshops.

Another interdisciplinary idea is to offer free workshops to the clients of another professional. For example, we could expand Kovacs' example and suggest workshops that might be offered to clients of tax preparers or accountants in their offices. Such topics might include "Why Spending Gets Out of Hand," "Resolving Money Differences: A

Workshop for Partners," and "Getting Organized to Reduce Taxtime Stress." Tax agency owner Ron Dannenberg suggested stress management workshops for tax preparers and a support group for the partners of preparers who are often casualties of the pressures of "tax season."[3]

Psychologist-author Sandra Haber routinely uses professional waiting rooms for psychotherapy workshops. For example, she has conducted a number of workshops for cancer patients in the waiting rooms of surgeons and oncologists and has addressed a new mothers' group on sleeping problems in newborns in the waiting room of a pediatric practice. This latter workshop could also be offered at a neighborhood playgroup, early childcare center, or children's clothing or furniture store.

As President of Psychologists in Independent Practice of the APA, Elaine Rodino worked on creating a workshop for training dentists and psychologists on practice benefits of understanding the psychological issues affecting dental patients. Issues such as TMD, bruxism, bulimia, dental anxiety and dental phobia, and self-image after tooth loss overlap both psychology and dentistry. These are issues that translate into workshops that can be held in dental offices for dental patients or presented at conferences for dentists or psychologists. Workshops can also be given to dental students at dental schools.

Key Advice On Workshops

Psychologist Neil Massoth[4] suggests that mental health therapists

> . . . look at opportunities outside of the 'traditional' role. . . . In addition to looking at job opportunities outside of your office or clinic (e.g. in industry, etc), don't overlook opportunities within your practice office doing things other than traditional psychotherapy. Some examples: groups for men; helping families deal with dementia. . . . Use your expertise; everyone has some.

Marketing Your Talk or Workshop

1. Select a host for your talk. This can be a large group, such as a synagogue or church, health club or yoga center; a specific neighborhood business, such as a sport shop or bookstore; or the premises of another professional, such as a pediatrician or surgeon.

2. Tie your topic into the interests of the members of the organization or patrons of the shop. In cases such as a synagogue or church, a number of topics are appropriate because the patrons are there with the usual problems of everyday life (including health, parenting, meeting a mate, and so on). In the case of the neighborhood bookstore, you might tie your topic into the subject matter of a book or series of books

they would like to feature (or it could even be a more generic topic for would-be writers such as overcoming writer's block or maximizing creativity). For specialized stores (e.g., sports shop) you will want to tie your talk into that specialty, such as "The Magic of Exercise," "Developing a Winning Attitude," or "The Psychology of Teambuilding." Obviously, workshops and talks in professional offices need to directly relate to the work of that professional; divorce-related issues would work for a lawyer whereas dental anxiety would be appropriate for dentists.

3. A month before the talk is to be given, print up flyers announcing the talk and ask the store owner (or professional) for help in distribution and marketing. Ask if he or she is willing to take out an ad in the local paper to announce your talk (since you are not being paid, this is a reasonable request), or if he or she already has a running ad, ask if it could be modified to feature information on your upcoming talk.

4. Write a press release (the "how to" appears in chapter 15) and send it to your local newspaper. If the host of your event already has an ad in this paper, mention it in your cover letter. (It makes those at the paper more likely to pay attention to it.) Ask to be placed on the community calendar, a standard feature in such newspapers.

5. Write a pitch letter (see chapter 15) directed toward the editor of the community paper or the individual who covers features such as the one you are offering. Check the masthead of the newspaper for names and addresses. Your pitch letter will tie your talk into other events that are significant to the reader and announce that you are available to be interviewed for an article. Enclose a copy of your flyer and invite the newspaper staff to attend your talk or workshop. If you have a fact sheet on your topic, enclose that too.

6. When any of your announcements, articles, or ads are printed in the newspaper, make copies of them and use them in future marketing ventures.

7. Consider handing out a brief two-page questionnaire after your workshop or talk. Invite comments on your workshop. Rave reviews can then be used in future marketing work. On the second page of your questionnaire, ask if people are interested in future workshops that you offer. They can list their names and addresses so that you can begin to compile a marketing list of people who enjoy your work and would be interested in future offerings.

8. Remember to distribute flyers, business cards, brochures, relevant reprints of articles, and resource lists to each attendee at your speech or workshop. Depending on your budget, consider the polished and professional look of placing your handouts in the pocket of an

8½ inch by 11 inch folder and stapling your business card to the front of the folder.

9. If possible, leave extra time at the end of your talk or workshop so that individuals in the audience can come up and speak with you privately. This private, one on one, time need only take a few minutes, but it sends the message that you are approachable. This creates a more personal and memorable connection beyond that of an ordinary workshop leader or speaker.

10. If your speech or workshop is educational (e.g., parenting, stress reduction, or smoking cessation), consider using promotional giveaways that audience members will save and use. Examples of such giveaways are buttons, pens, Post-it® Notes, and refrigerator magnets. Each can be imprinted with a memorable "tip" and your office phone number. Examples of such tips would be "Did you hug your child today?" or "Stressful things are usually little things." Giveaway items can be found under "promotionals" in the Yellow Pages of your telephone directory.

11. Promotionals can also be effective with professional audiences. For example, Laurie Kolt[5] developed courtesy cards for nontherapist professionals that have an educational paragraph on "When to Refer." The card of course also had her name, address, and phone number.

Tote bags, coffee mugs, and mouse pads imprinted with "When the road of life takes a tough turn, a psychologist can help" are promotionals that are used by the Psychologists in Independent Practice to market psychology (Figure 13.1). These items are used by psychologists and given to colleagues as holiday gifts.

Key Advice
Montreal psychologist, Barbara Wainrib notes

When changes in the (Canadian) health care system caused most of my referrals to move away, I focused on my own personal interest—women's issues. I offered a course in women and mid-life at the YWCA and only 6 women signed up. However, on the day it started, an article about me and the course appeared in the newspaper. Sixty women showed up, and we had to run two programs. . . . After that, a group of 20 of them formed a women's group that met privately at my office for the following year. For several years after that, I gave many such workshops in the different areas and suburbs of the cities and as my name became known I was asked to do a 11 growing number of public speaking 'gigs' locally and nationally. While the workshops and speeches do not necessarily afford direct referrals, they familiarize people with your name, so when they are looking for a therapist and are offered several suggestions, if they

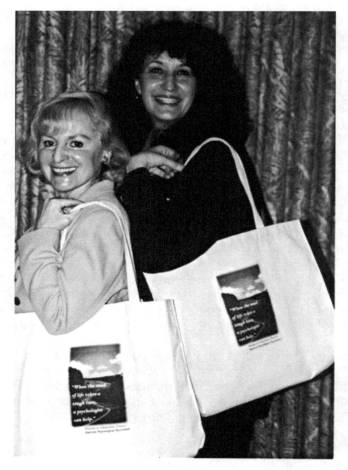

FIGURE 13.1   Promotional tote bags. (Courtesy of Dr. Elaine Rodino [left] and Dr. Sandra Huber [right].)

recognize yours they feel more comfortable in calling you . . . (also) one should never overlook the importance of a single referral. I sometimes trace referrals back to their original source and a single good referral can lead to hundreds of others.[6]

NOTES

[1] Personal communication, January 10, 2000.
[2] Personal communication, April 13, 1999.

[3] Personal communication, January 10, 1997.
[4] Personal communication, January 15, 2000.
[5] Personal communication, January 7, 1999.
[6] B. Wainrib, personal communication, January 20, 1999.

REFERENCES

Kalish, K. (1999). *How to give a terrific presentation.* Washington, DC: Kalish Communications.
Kalish, K. (1999). Ten steps for speech preparation. Available: Kalish Communications, 2120 S. Street NW, Washington, DC 20008.
Stuttard, M. (1997). *The power of public speaking.* New York: Barron's Educational Series.

Chapter 14

Web Listings and Basic Web Pages

Thinking about a Web site? Whether you are technologically challenged or technologically sophisticated you can have a Web-site presence that will serve to supplement your practice and provide the public and other professionals with information about yourself and your services. Believe it or not, you do not even need to own a computer to add a bit of cyberspace to your marketing armament.

SIMPLE WEB PRESENCE

Even if you do not own a computer, you can have a basic Web presence by being mentioned on another Web-site. For example, psychologist Don Franklin[1] has a Web site that includes a National Directory of Psychologists. The National Register of Providers of Psychology also provides a Web-site listing of psychologists. The American Mental Health Alliance (AMHA), an interdisciplinary group of psychotherapists, is in the process of creating a Web-site directory of affiliates. Your professional organization on a local, state, and national level is likely to be developing a Web site that will be able to list your practice information.

Another way of having a Web presence is by consulting to a specialty Web site. One of the authors (S.H.) is a consultant to an exercise and dieting Web site and receives a large number of media referrals each month asking her to respond to the psychological aspects of fitness. Kate Hays notes that although she does not have a Web site, her professional information is linked in with two other Web sites, giving her practice added visibility. "While I don't have a Web-site of my own, the dental pamphlet is on the Web . . . and . . . the Canadian International Marathon has a Web site and they're about to post a page on the Psyching Team for the marathon that I'm in the midst of creating—along with a bio of me."[2]

WEB-SITE DEVELOPMENT

Your own Web site with Web pages can supplement your practice and provide the public and other professionals with information about you and your services. A Web site is a collection of one or more Web pages that link together to make a presentation. You can share your ideas, educate people, and market your specialization. You can connect your Web pages with professional organizations and create links to other sites that will give you a marketing advantage. Since the Internet has no time zones or geographic boundaries, it is a convenient way to reach a larger, more diverse audience either at home or at work. It is generally recognized that a Web-site supplements, rather than substitutes for, brochures, flyers, ads, and other marketing materials. A Web-site can be an economical way of advertising and conducting e-commerce, although Dick Anderson[3] of AdVentures notes that, in the beginning, therapists should view their Web site as income enhancing rather than income producing.

GUIDELINES FOR BEGINNERS

As with any new venture, a Web site takes time to plan, develop, and promote. One way you can begin to get familiar with the Internet and the Web is by browsing through cyberspace and looking at what others have done with their Web sites. While browsing, consider what you want to do with your Web site, who you want to reach, and what kinds of information you want on your site.

Determine what your goals are. A Web-site can be used in many different ways. A basic Web site should contain information about your practice, office address, phone and e-mail contact (if available). In chapter 17 we will discuss more sophisticated uses for your Web site.

EXAMPLE OF A BASIC WEB SITE

An example of a Web site can be seen in Figure 14.1.

Psychological Services of Raleigh, P.A.

Mary Kilburn, Ph.D.
Licensed Psychologist

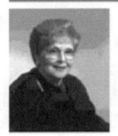

- About Mary Kilburn, Ph.D.
- Counseling & Psychotherapy
- Stopping Smoking
- Location
- Insurance and Payments
- Getting Started
- Links to Useful Sites

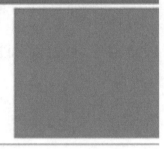

Email: marykilburn@mindspring.com

Telephone with secure answering machine: 919-781-5162

Off the Beltline near NORTH HILLS SHOPPING CENTER.
Exit at I-440 and Six Forks Road (SOUTH).

Barrett Square I

4016 Barrett Drive, Suite 104

Raleigh, North Carolina 27609-6623

FIGURE 14.1   Example of a basic Web site.

Personal Experience

Mary Kilburn, psychologist, notes

> I chose to use a preexisting template available through 'Hometown at
> AOL.' . . . It was up within a couple of hours, ready for connection to other
> sites such as 'Psychologists USA.'. . . Since I used a pre-established tem-
> plate, there's little freedom for either true creativity or expansion. This,
> however, is inspiring me to move on to something considerably more
> sophisticated in the future . . . (and) I have received phone calls and
> emails from both media (an interest of mine) and potential patients. As
> an interesting note, my experience with patients who followed through
> on our initial contact is that they were more often non-managed care
> payers as contrasted with other referral sources. This seems to make
> sense in that persons seeking insurance or managed care reimburse-
> ment would likely be channeled through their in-house directories or
> gatekeepers, so that those doing an open search on the Internet may
> be more open to direct pay for services. . . . Last but not least, develop-
> ing a Web-site can provide an ongoing outlet which is both creative
> and fun![4]

HOW DO YOU GET A WEB SITE?

The first decision you need to make is whether your Web site will be professionally developed or do-it-yourself. Note that in both cases, you need to get a Web site that works for you and the people you are trying to reach. You will need to decide on the text, write it in a Web-site–friendly manner, and make decisions about design and layout. With this as a common denominator, here are some of the considerations of a professionally developed site versus a do-it yourself site.

Professionally Developed Web Site

- You do not need to learn the more technical details of Web construction.
- You will be billed by the hour for the time it takes to create your site or you will be given a per page price. Typically, the fee for hiring the services of a Web designer to build the site for you is several hundred dollars.
- You are dependent on your Web professional to make a changes to your site that may reduce the frequency and quality of your efforts to keep your site up to date, removing, adding, and updating information.
- Often, a professionally produced site has a more professional and polished appearance.
- Cross listing your Web page to other sites may involve an extra fee.

Do-It-Yourself Web Site

- The site can be developed at no or low cost.
- There is a computer skills learning curve involved. The amount you will have to learn will vary according to how elaborate your site is.
- You can use your existing software to create a home page, which is the first page of your Web site. This is often provided by your Internet server; it is user friendly and tends to reduce the amount of technical details you have to master.
- This may involve the purchase of software. Web software is also available through office productivity software, such as Microsoft Office 97 or 2000. The most you should pay for professional Web authoring software is about $100.
- Creating your own site can often result in a more up-to-date site because you have the skills to make changes at no extra cost.
- Doing it yourself will involve additional time following development of the Web page to cross list your site so people can find it.

WHAT ABOUT THE COSTS OF A WEB SITE?

As previously noted there are many services that include Web-site space as a free part of their service. The Internet service provider one uses (AOL, AT&T, Earthlink, Mindspring, etc.) usually has free space available to subscribers. There are also many sites that give free space in exchange for advertising space on your pages.

For a professionally developed site, you can expect the approximate costs to break out like this:

- Domain registration. Every domain (www.Your Name) needs to register to be on the Web.
- A one-time set-up fee charged by Web servers
- Per page charge
- Web hosting charge
- Maintenance fees monitor site, make changes (additions, deletions, etc.). Maintenance usually includes keeping track of the number of visitors to your Web site. Maintenance also has to include an ongoing effort to find more effective ways to make your site more visible through off-line marketing, reciprocal links, and search engines. There is a basic maintenance fee for small sites with few changes during the year and a higher fee if you add pages regularly or make changes often.
- Total costs vary depending on how complex your site is to design and maintain. Generally speaking, an attractive site an be developed for a few hundred dollars and a site with minimal changes should have a similar annual fee.

HOW DO PEOPLE FIND YOUR WEB SITE?

Whether you pay someone to do this for you or decide to do it yourself, it should be clear that your Web site will not serve your purposes as a marketing tool if the people you are trying to reach fail to find it. Even if you are hiring a Web master to maintain your site and list it on search engines, it behooves you to be an informed consumer. The simplest links are with other mental health organizations or related Web sites. Psychology Information Online offers other psychologists an opportunity to publish articles on its Web site with a byline and a link back to their practice Web site. PsychologistsUSA is a free service that links the Web sites of licensed psychologists, provided they link back to the PsychologistsUSA main page. Reciprocal arrangements for linking Web sites will continue to become available.

More typically, people will find your site using search engines such as Dogpile, Excite, Google, Infoseek, Lycos and Yahoo, for which they have put in a key word, such as "psychotherapist." Many search engines offer you the option of listing your site with them. It makes their work easier if you go to them, so there are mutual benefits. Search engines then display sites in a particular order. This order is very important, notes Tim Platt of InFoMed Consulting, because most people only scan the first screen of search engine hits, as they are called.[5] If your site appears too far down the list, no one will ever get to it or to you in their search. There are businesses that specialize in getting the word out to search engines and other sites for you. They generally do this by submitting your Internet address to hundreds of places at once.

You can improve your odds, according to Tim Platt,[6] of being found both online and offline by adding "metatags" to your Web pages. These are internal, under the hood, resources that provide information about your page but do not show on your Web pages. You should discuss metatags with your Web designer so that they are specific to your service.

You can list key words and all the synonyms you want in the links so that search engines find them. One approach to finding the right key words in designing your site is to ask prospective users what words they would try. For example, if your specialty is eating disorders, you might find out that John or Jane Q. Public is most likely to look under "dieting" or "weight loss," not "eating disorder," so the former terms would be important key words.

ADVICE FROM PRACTITIONERS

I believe that the potential of the Internet for the identification and provision of new forms of psychological help is far, far greater than we can even imagine. It would be a great mistake to ignore that potential.[7]

My advice would be to recognize that the strong trend is for potential consumers to continue to become more computer literate. This means that potential clients and referral sources will be doing more research and communication online in the days, weeks, months and years to come. Having a Web site is a way of connecting with potential patients and referral sources. It will some day be similar to having a listing in the yellow pages.[8]

I have a Web site, and it gets me expert witness work from across the country. Martin Williams,[9] psychologist, reports, I realize that not everyone has an expert witness practice, but a Web site can also get you psychotherapy business or serve as an educational asset for your existing patients. . . . I think it's time for even the most technophobic of us to realize that having a Web-site might be the new equivalent of having a listing in the telephone book. From this point of view, it's not a question of whether having your own Web-site is good for business, it's more a question of whether not having one is bad for business.

This is only the beginning of a new adventure for the mixture of psychology and technology. Fink (1999, p. xxi) notes that "as technology develops, improving our ability to connect in cyberspace, humans will continue to adapt to life online. We are witnessing the merging of two provocative and powerful forces: psychology and technology. I call this merging psychotechnology."

In chapter 17 we will discuss more elaborate and advanced Web activities, including virtual groups, interactive Web sites, online counseling, and e-zines.

NOTES

[1] Personal communication, January 22, 2000.
[2] K. Hayes, personal communication, May 20, 1999.
[3] Personal communication, May 1, 1999.
[4] Personal communication, June 18, 1999.
[5] Personal communication, February 10, 2000.
[6] Personal communication, February 10, 2000.
[7] R. Fox, personal communication, May 9, 1999.
[8] L. Beer, personal communication, May 10, 1999.
[9] Personal communication, March 3, 1999.

REFERENCE

Fink, J. (1999). *How to use computers and cyberspace in the clinical practice of psychotherapy*. Northvale, NJ: Jason Aronson.

Part VI

Advanced Tools of the Trade

Chapter 15

Press Releases, Pitch Letters, and Authoring a Book

Worried about tooting your own horn? Don't be. Think of it as creating news that can help you give psychology away.

PRESS RELEASES

A press release is the basic communication tool of public relations. It is a simple statement of who, what, when, where, how, and why. Michael Levine, author of *Guerrilla PR,* (1993) notes that the *Wall Street Journal* reports that 90% of its coverage originates with companies making their own announcements, most of which are sent to the newspaper in the form of a press release.

In writing your own press release, make the title and lead sentence intriguing. The first and second paragraphs then explain the "news." Your wrap-up paragraph gives the details of the event and how the reader can get further information. Usually, a press release is one page, or at most two pages, long.

Details of Writing a Press Release

- The words "For Immediate Release" appear on the upper left corner of the page.
- The date the material is sent out appears on the upper right corner of the page.

- Contact information appears at the top right of the first page and includes your name and phone numbers.
- The heading of the press release is centered on the page and followed by a few paragraphs of text.
- The symbols ### appear at the end of the text to signify the end of the release.

Marketing with a Press Release

If you are announcing an event, send your press release 10 days ahead of time for a daily paper. If you are marketing to a small community newspaper with a monthly distribution, call to ascertain the appropriate time frame. Often, it can be as long as 6 weeks ahead of publication. After sending your press release, call the newspaper and have a brief follow-up conversation to be sure your item has arrived. If your release is printed, send a thank you note to the reporter or editor who is responsible for the pick up.

Example of a Press Release

Figure 15.1 presents a sample press release.

Best Advice

The best advice for writing a press release comes from Kelly Cunningham, owner of ImPRessions, a public relations firm. She states that "Reporters receive so many press releases that it is imperative that you make yours as interesting and succinct as possible."[1]

PITCH LETTERS

Closely related to a press release is a pitch letter sent to print media experts to suggest a story. It combines many of the features of a press release but also suggests to the reporter a story angle and an individual to contact. In your marketing plan, you can develop a roster of local or national reporters with whom you regularly communicate through the use of pitch letters. In each letter, you describe an "angle" for a story that is often tied to the newsbreaking item of the day, provide information on why psychology is relevant to the story, and then offer to make yourself available for further comment.

Note that pitch letters are more personalized than are press releases, are addressed to a particular individual, and have overall a more

Today's Date

CONTACT: Jane Albright, C.S.W.
000-555-0000

DEPRESSION NEED NOT KEEP YOU DOWN!

Jane Albright, a New York City psychotherapist and associate professor at New York University, will give a free talk for the public called "Depression Need Not Keep You Down: Techniques to Manage, Cope and Conquer." The talk is cosponsored by Hamilton Hospital and will be offered on Wed. night, Oct. 14 at 7:30 PM at the hospital clinic at 1440 Jorame Ave., New York City.

A recent article in *The New York Times* notes that depression may be a useful response helping people to disengage from hopeless situations that are simple not working. This "Darwinian perspective" is a more positive way of understanding this mental health problem and affects 17 million Americans each year and 10% of the population.

Depression occurs when feelings of extreme sadness or despair last for 2 weeks or longer and begin to interfere with the activities of daily living including patterns of work, sleeping, and eating. Depression can abe conquered as exemplified by baseball champion Mark Maguire,* who openly discusses his experience with depression. "I was having all kinds of relationship problems. I didn't know what love was all about. I had four brothers and no sisters. We never talked about it. You're never taught" These are how feelings are. It's like you're waling into a dark room and just feeling blindly around." Maguire credits his 4 years of psychotherapy with understanding and overcoming his depression. "It took failure to understand myself," he notes.

In her talk, Albright will review how psychotherapy helps people recover from depression and how the feeling of losing can be turned into one of winning. Jane Albright's talk will be offered at Hamilton Hospital on October 14 at 7:30 PM. The hospital is located at 1440 Jorame Ave., New York City. The talk will be free of charge.

* From P. Reilly, "The Good Father," *Sports Illustrated*, September 7, 1998, p. 38.

FIGURE 15.1. Example of a press release.

personal style. A pitch letter paints a picture for the editor or media person. It may include key messages and provides contact information and background material as well as a suggested person to interview. Figure 15.2 provides an example of a pitch letter.

MARKETING WITH PRINT MEDIA

National Days and Events

In public relations, as in life, timing is everything. Keep your eyes open for national days and events to tie in your marketing efforts. Some examples of these events are shown in Figure 15.3.

In addition, your local newspapers will respond to pitch ideas about local events that often occur at times that are different from the national event. Typical examples include cancer and health-related walks or runs that are dependent on the weather in your region. Additionally, the media may be open to your input if you tie your psychological expertise in with a popular book, first-run movie, or a trauma or natural disaster that effects a local resident or family.

Shaping Your Press Release or Pitch

It is helpful to remember that each event can have a direct pitch (the psychology of the event itself) or an indirect pitch. For examples, National Secretary's Day can be about the importance of acknowledging helpful business relationships or it can propose remedies for problems such as anger or disrespect in a boss. A June pitch on graduation can address the joy of moving on and completing one's education, or it can address the anxiety of leaving the safe shelter of a school. A June marriage pitch can focus on the magic and wonder of a wedding or the difficulty of being single. National TV Turnoff Week can focus on fun alternatives to television or it can offer ways to communicate more effectively with your children. If you are imaginative and creative, you will never run out of newsworthy angles to pitch.

AUTHORING A BOOK

So you want to write a book? Good idea and more doable that you might think. There is probably no better way to get name recognition, credibility, and expertise with a wide audience. Be aware, however, that although authoring a book can serve as a powerful marketing

Today's Date

Name of reporter

Medical Health Column

Name of Newspaper

Dear Ms./Mr. Name of Reporter:

On (give date) millions of Americans will tune in their TV sets to watch the Winter Olympics. Viewers will admire the discipline, perseverance, and courage that these athletes demonstrate, and many will wonder how to connect the performance of these champions with sport-related activities in their own lives. "Sports psychology" is a new burgeoning field of applied psychology that can help all individuals—from the Little League coach to the amateur tennis enthusiast—to enjoy and enhance their game. In conjunction with the Olympic Event, I'd like to suggest a story on how sports psychology can help the ordinary American bring fun and health into their lives.

Sport psychology has two definitions that are important to your readers. The first, and the one that most people are familiar with, is the psychological factors that influence success in a sport. Example of this include stress management, goal setting, and mental imagery. The second, less known, definition is the effect that a sport or regular exercise has on individual functioning. This includes improving self-esteem, reducing depression and anxiety, and increasing mental and emotional functioning.

As a licensed psychologist and an expert in sport psychology, I can discuss these factors with you and translate the scientific findings into practical tips. I would like to offer you an interview to discuss this material further.

I look forward to speaking with you.

Sincerely,

John Doe, Ph.D.

FIGURE 15.2 Example of pitch letter.

tool, book writing is a long-term, intensive effort and definitely not for everyone. Psychotherapist Ofer Zur cautions, "Books, which take years to write, generally make neither much money nor generate a large referral base" (2000, p. 29). Of course many psychotherapists disagree and have found authoring a book to be personally gratifying and a passport to opportunities for public speaking, workshop presentation, and other opportunities that ultimately generate a substantial client base.

MARK YOUR CALENDAR!

February
Eating Disorder Awareness Week
Wise Health Consumer Month
American Heart Month
National Girls and Women in Sports Day

March
National Nutrition Month
Children and Healthcare Week

April
National Child Abuse Prevention Month
National Cancer Control Month
National Public Health Week

May
National Mental Health Awareness Month
National Anxiety Disorders Screening Day
National Suicide Awareness Week
National Running and Fitness Week
National Employee Health and Fitness Day
National Senior Health and Fitness Day
Older Americans Month

September
Prostate Cancer Awareness Month
National Cholesterol Education Month

October
Breast Cancer Awareness Month
National Mammography Day
Mental Illness Awareness Week
National Depression Screening Day
Family Health Month
National Heart Walk—American Heart Association
National Health Education Week
National Youth Health Awareness Day
Child Health Month

November
National Alzheimer's Awareness Month
Great American Smoke Out

FIGURE 15.3 Example of key dates in 1998. (From *The Practice Directorate*. New York: American Psychological Association.)

In deciding whether or not you should author a book, consider some of these personal musings from psychologist-author Barbara Wainrib:

> So—why write a book? Obviously there has to be some reinforcement. This can either be in the process or the product.
>
> Reinforcement in the process might include a sense of achievement in either the researching and interviewing, the writing, or the connection to the audience. Sometimes, the reinforcement is simply from the sense of connection and shared creativity with one's writing partner.
>
> Reinforcement from the product includes a gratification related to money, contentment with oneself, pride (or narcissistic feeding), connections for other people, sense of achievement, sense of moving into some new area of expertise or respect, passion about the subject or sense of giving new ideas or reorganized ideas to the audience.[2]

If your personal soul searching gives you a green light on book writing, then here are some useful informational items that will move you towards successful authorship.

Professional Books

Professional books are published through professional publishing houses. Generally, these publishers can be found in the exhibit area at most major professional meetings, or you can simply look at the professional books you use to decide which publisher might be most appropriate for your book.

If you are interested in writing a professional book, call the publishing house for a copy of their author's guidelines. This will be a written document that will spell out the proposal and writing process. Discuss your ideas with the representative from the publishing house. Professional publishers are usually very friendly and willing to discuss a potential book. They are always looking for new and interesting material and offer valuable suggestions about how to frame your topic. Typically, you will be asked to submit a summary of the book, the chapter titles and content, and a sample first chapter. You can follow the author's guidelines for preparing this part of the submission or ask the publishing representative to send you a sample copy that you use as a guide.

If your manuscript is accepted, you can expect to discuss the possibilities of an advance (sometimes yes, sometimes no, usually minimal), royalty rate (usually 10% on initial sales and rising to 15% for a strong seller), and manuscript due date. You will be sent a contract in which all of the agreed upon details are presented in writing.

Remember that professional books rarely generate significant amounts of income. What it can do is provide you with speaking, teaching, and referral opportunities.

Trade Books

If you decide you want to write a book for the public, you will be working with a trade publishing house. With trade books, it is usually helpful to work with a literary agent. Although libraries and bookstores have books listing literary agents, you will meet with greater success if you find an agent through personal contact or through a colleague who has published a trade book. The agent's name is also likely to appear in the acknowledgment section of a book; so that, books that are on a topic similar to yours may be a resource for this information.

Literary agents typically receive 15% of all book profits; often this is money well-earned. In addition to selling your book to a publishing house, they also negotiate for the highest possible advance and arbitrate the proposed contract. One of the authors (SH) of this book had a trade book published that was remaindered (went out of print) after the first year. Because the agent was diligent, the rights to the book reverted back to the authors, who then updated, revised, and published a revised edition of the book with another publishing house. Needless to say, the intricate mechanics of all this could not have been accomplished without the tutelage of a good agent.

In trade publication, there is usually advance money. At times this can be quite sizable. Frequently, this is the only real money to be made on a book. The way this works is that you will be offered an advance for your book, part of which is given to you upon signing, part on the delivery of the manuscript, and part on publication. The profits of the book are then used to pay back the advance that the publishers gave you. The author receives royalties only after the advance is paid back.

In trade publications, you are often expected to work with a writer. At times, the publishing house will pay for the writer. Most often, particularly with beginning authors, you will be expected to hire and pay for the writer. Often you will pay the writer out of pocket for the proposal. If the book is sold, the advance money will usually cover the rest of the writer's fee and (hopefully) give you some profit. Remember, too, that the advance money will include the agent's fee.

The guidelines in the box can get you started. They were contributed by literary agent Faith Hamlin of Sanford Greenberger Associates in New York City.

Seven Questions People Most Frequently Ask Literary Agents

1. How do I know if I have a salable book idea? Do research on the subject. Check bookstores, *Books in Print,* Amazon.com. Is your idea really new? Is there a large enough audience for your book (several million minimum)? Are you an expert in this field? Have you done research on the topic? Has your theory been tested? Do you teach or speak on the subject or have a media platform?

2. What does an agent need to see to be enthusiastic about my project? It is not advisable to write the whole book before you try to sell it. A proposal works much better, and it leaves room for a change in format or focus. A good proposal contains an overview, a complete biography of the author, a table of contents, chapter descriptions, a section on who will buy the book and why, and a thorough analysis of the most competitive titles. Why is your book better than the books out there? You'll also need a sample chapter or two. There are a number of books available on how to write a proposal. Consulting these is a must. Many a good idea is lost in a bad proposal.

3. How do I find an agent? How do I choose an agent? If you have friends who write books, ask them if they are happy with their agent. Look in the acknowledgments of favorite, related books, and consult books on how to find an agent. Choose an agent with whom you feel comfortable, one who is willing to answer lots of questions and work on your proposal with you. Look for someone who has demonstrated expertise in your fields of interest and who therefore has strong editor contacts in major publishing houses. Ask for the titles of books the agent has sold and have a look at them.

4. How do I contact an agent? Write a strong query letter describing your project, say why this idea is salable and why you are the person to write the book. Be sure to emphasize your credentials—degrees, experience, awards, media experience, workshops, lectures, and publishing credits. Your credentials and visibility in the field are critical to marketing you and your book. Offer to send your proposal (or enclose it, if it's not more than about 15 pages). Make your letter succinct and inviting, very specific but not too long (1–2 pages). Be sure to enclose a stamped, self-addressed envelope (S.A.S.E.). You may send your letter to a number of agents simultaneously, but let each of them know you are

doing so. You should follow up by telephone, if you haven't heard anything in about three weeks, or if you receive interest from one of the agents.

5. Why do I need an agent? It is hard to find an appropriate publisher and editor and negotiate the deal on your own. Some publishers won't even accept submissions from you without an agent. The agent becomes your business partner. He/she promotes you in a way you can't promote yourself—preserving the delicate relationship between you and your publisher. This allows you to concentrate on the creative aspects of writing. In addition, the agent helps you shape your proposal in order to realize the book's fullest potential. Publishers prefer to deal with agents because they don't have to explain everything to the author.

Your agent has contacts at all major publishing houses and may send your proposal to several publishers simultaneously. This gives the agent the possibility of auctioning the book for the best deal, both in money and other terms. She then negotiates the contract and markets the rights not granted to the publisher—foreign and film, for example. The agent explains everything to you along the way, stays involved throughout the life of the book and mediates any disputes. The agent also is your main supporter and champion in areas of sales, advertising and publicity. Should the editor leave the company, the publisher fold or your book be rejected when you deliver it, you need someone in your corner. The agent is the constant in an ever-changing publishing world.

6. How do I know if I need to work with a writer? If you are a busy person and/or writing doesn't come easily to you, get a writer. If your book is meant for a popular audience, an experienced writer can write in a way that will reach that market. A good agent will help you find an appropriate and compatible writer. The project will be professional and you will meet your deadline. Be sure you have a collaboration agreement in writing that is signed by all parties before work begins.

7. What will a book do for my career? You will become better known in your field, will be more likely to be asked to speak, lecture, comment to the media and be promoted if you teach. If you have a practice you will be more likely to attract clients. Other professionals will recommend your book to their patients in order to help them understand their problems. (From Hamlin [1998]. Used with permission.)

Self-Publishing

Self-publishing is when you pay for your own book to be published. It is executed through a self-publishing house. Typical costs are (approximately) $10,000 for the first 1,000 books. You can also use the self-publishing house to hire a public relations expert to promote your book. The fee here is variable and depends on the number and type of tasks you are requesting.

Self-publishing is an option that can be considered for both professional and trade books. According to Elliot Wolf,[3] owner of Wolf-Wilke Press, self-publishing offers two distinct advantages to traditional publishing. The first advantage is that of control. A self-publishing company is your employee and will publish your materials according to your wishes. The second advantage of self-publishing can be financial If you are ready, willing, and able to promote your book, all of the profits belong to you. This method can be very successful if and only if you are actively on the road and able to market your book yourself. This means that you will need to have many speaking or workshop engagements, will arrange to have the books shipped to the site, and will have an individual on site to take credit cards, checks, or cash and monitor the book sales. Extra books will need to be shipped back. You can also write articles referring to your book and send out sample books for editorial review.

A few mental health professionals will do very well with the self-publishing approach, but for the majority of our readers we recommend (at least for the first time book experience) going a more traditional route.

Final Note

Although self-publication requires the most intensive marketing efforts, it is wise to remember that you, the author, need to be involved in marketing your book no matter how it is published. Steve Brody,[4] psychologist-author notes that ". . . expectations can be unrealistic." A 14-city tour to promote his book was successful but did not result in a best-seller. Steve noted that laziness was a factor.

> I was riding on my past successes, and in order to pull such a venture like this off, I needed to be willing to push this new stone up the hill . . . something I no longer really wanted to do. Again, you've got to be willing and eager to sacrifice your time and energy for 'the cause.' You need to be honest with yourself and ask yourself if you really have the passion, commitment, and emotional and financial reserves to go the distance. If you don't, there's no shame in admitting that to yourself, and proceeding accordingly. You need the emotional intelligence to know yourself and what you're willing and able to do at this stage of your life.[5]

NOTES

[1] Personal communication, June 1, 1999.
[2] Personal communication, May 20, 1999.
[3] Personal communication, January 24, 2000.
[4] Personal communication, March 12, 1999.
[5] Personal communication, March 12, 1999.

REFERENCES

Hamlin, F. (August, 1998). Seven questions people most frequently ask literary agents. New York: Sanford J. Greenburger Associates.

Levine, M. (1993). *Guerrilla PR*. New York: HarperCollins.

Wainrib, B., & Haber, S. (2000). *Men, women and prostate cancer: A medical and psychological guide*. Oakland, CA: New Harbinger.

Zur, O. (2000, Winter). Marketing 101. *Independent Practitioner, 20,* 28–31.

Chapter 16

Interviewing for Print, Radio, and Television

I f you are interested in contributing to public education, are intrigued by the idea of communicating to a wide audience, and desire widespread name recognition, then newspapers, magazines, radio, and television are media to market your message. Although you may never be the new Dr. Joyce Brothers, media exposure can generate familiarity and credibility for you, your service, and your product.

In this chapter we will describe overall pointers that apply to all forms of the media followed by some tips that are unique to each communication modality.

GENERAL SUGGESTIONS FOR PRINT, RADIO, AND TELEVISION INTERVIEWS OR APPEARANCES

Content

Be sure to find out what the interviewer is looking for. What information do they want? Are they looking for an expert who can express a particular position on an issue or one who can describe many aspects of a problem? Will you be primarily educating the audience (news-type show) or entertaining the audience (some daytime interview shows)?

Audience

What are the demographics of the readers, listeners, or viewers; in other words, who is the audience? This includes age, gender, socioeconomic

147

level, educational level, as well as section of the country (urban, rural, etc.). An interview on relationships will be very different for *Seventeen* magazine than it is for *Modern Maturity*. The topic of physical attractiveness would be presented differently on CNN than it is on Oprah Winfrey. Familiarity with your audience will help you shape a more useful message.

Details

Timing

When will the interview take place? For news-breaking stories, the reporter may request an immediate response, whereas a TV show will usually have a specific day and time already set aside. A magazine will typically request an interview that can be responded to within a week. Find out if the interviewer is "on deadline" to determine the degree of flexibility and to help you respond appropriately. At a minimum, we suggest that you never respond immediately to an interview request. Rather, arrange to call the interviewer back in 15 minutes to give yourself time to gather your thoughts about the topic.

Location

Print media interviews are often conducted on the telephone. Radio interviews are frequently conducted on the telephone and sometimes are conducted from the radio station. Some television interviews can be conducted in your office; others are conducted at the television station.

Payment

Unless you are a media personality or member of the actors union, there is typically no payment for any type of media work.

Perks

If you request it, you may be sent a copy of the magazine or interview or be given a tape of your radio or television appearance.

Preparation

No matter what the medium, you will need time to prepare your comments for the interview. Media consultants advise that you write down the three major points that you want to make; these are called your "talking points." Television interviews rarely allow for more than these three points, though you may have more latitude in a lengthier radio interview or print interview.

Translate your talking points into audience-friendly pieces of information. These are called sound bites. For example, if one point for a parenting interview is "Parents should use positive reinforcement rather than negative reinforcement to elicit optimal behaviors in their children," then an appropriate talking point, phrased as a sound bite would be "Parents should remember: Rewards Work!" You will more likely be quoted directly with these "catchy" phrases rather than long, drawn out explanations. This is true for all media outlets.

SPECIFIC TIPS: PRINT, RADIO, AND TELEVISION

Print

- Tip 1. If the journalist has contacted you because of a breaking story, there may be an immediate deadline. If you get the message and have not returned the call within the hour, your interview has probably gone to another mental health professional. If you do contact the journalist immediately try not to be pressured into an immediate interview. First, ascertain whether you are familiar enough with the topic to give a response. If you are not, tell them your area(s) of expertise (for future reference) and then refer them to a knowledgeable colleague or to your local, state, or national psychotherapy association. If you the think the topic is within your area of expertise, ask to call them in 15 minutes so you can gather your thoughts.
- Tip 2. Print interviews that do not have immediate deadlines are often pleasant, comfortable, and casual. For example, in "lifestyle" interviews for magazines or newspapers, the journalist often works from his or her home as a freelancer and tends to have an unhurried, casual style. This frequently will lead to a positive interview experience. Just be sure to remember that "off the record" does not really exist. If you discuss your personal experience with a topic (divorce, children, etc.), it is part of the interview. Be sure to consider this long-term effect (you may see it in print!) before including it in the conversation.
- Tip 3. Most print interviews without immediate time constraints result in clear and complete explanation of psychological issues, so the journalist will be more likely to correctly reflect your opinions. Often, you will get to see or are read your portion of the article before it goes to print. Magazines routinely do this through the editing department, who will call, fax, or e-mail you your materials to verify your quotes. Newspapers most frequently, do not do this because of the time constraints.

Although some media trainers recommend that you ask for a copy in order to permit them to print your interview, we feel that this is most often a reflection of the policy of the newspaper or magazine, not a decision to be made by the reporter or author. If you are "difficult" to interview, they will interview someone else. You can ask to review the material before it is printed, but, generally speaking, clarity in sound bites is your ticket to accurate reporting.

- Tip 4. Be sure to spell your name and give your title and degrees and as much identifying information as possible. Remember that part of your goal is self-marketing. Consider the marketing implications of the following three citations: "According to Jane Smith, a couples psychotherapist in Boise, Idaho," "According to Jane Smith, a psychotherapist in Boise, Idaho," and "According to Jane Smith, psychotherapist."

Need we say more?

Radio

- Tip 1. In a radio interview, the key advantage is that you can be heard but not seen. Take advantage of this feature and have your talking points written down and with you, whether you do the interview at the radio station or from your home. These written points will help you stay focused and keep the interview on track.
- Tip 2. Many radio stations feature a call-in segment. In this case, the caller will sometimes ask questions that are relevant to your topic and will sometimes ask questions that are off the topic. Be sure you know how to "bridge" a question that you cannot or do not want to answer and return to your particular points. Examples of bridging a question to return to the topic at hand are: "But my experience is that," Follow an inappropriate comment or question with "A more important point is that," or, "What I really think is important is."
- Tip 3. Have the number of a mental health clinic or your local, state, or national psychotherapy association on hand, so that you have a referral suggestion if the person calling seems to have a more personal problem that needs immediate attention.

Television

- Tip 1. Television requires time management. If the interview is to be conducted at your office, discuss the timing with the booker and free up 1/2 hour before and 1/2 hour after the appointment time. The earlier time is used for your preparation; the later time is used for the crew to rearrange your furniture, dismantle the camera lighting, and exit your office. Note that news-breaking crews may need to cancel an interview if a different story takes precedence.

When the television appearance is scheduled at the studio, you will be asked to arrive early and wait (usually in the green room, which is almost never green). This down time is used to assemble the guests, arrange for your hair and makeup to be touched up, and view earlier segments of the show. The latter piece will help you anticipate your own interview. If you are on a panel, you can use this time to establish a rapport with the other individuals waiting to be interviewed. This rapport helps the on-air interview go smoothly.

- Tip 2. In television, appearance counts. Media experts advise wearing conservative clothing. Media trainer and expert Karen Kalish's (1999) favorite tips note that women's apparel should be a suit or dress with sleeves in a solid color of blue, gray, winter white, deep red, or purple with only plain jewelry. Women should also wear their usual makeup, without overdoing it. Men are advised to wear a solid color jacket, navy blue suit, or sport coat; pastel shirt; red or burgundy tie; polished shoes; and socks above the calf. No zig-zag patterns on shirts or ties that play tricks on the camera.

  If your interview is at a network TV station, makeup and hair will typically be done for you. If your interview is on a cable TV station or in your office, you will usually need to do your makeup and hair yourself. In this case, a bit of powder to the forehead, cheeks, or chin for both men and women will keep lights from reflecting off your face. The booker can tell you if grooming services will be provided.

- Tip 3. Remember and rehearse your three talking points. You will not be able to carry a cue card with you, so you need to know these points cold.

- Tip 4. Just before the interview begins, you will be hooked to a microphone, which will usually go on the jacket of your lapel. You will be asked to speak into the microphone. Rather than the usual counting of numbers, it is wiser to say "This is Jane Doe, psychotherapist. J-A-N-E D-O-E. Often there is a card printed with your name that will flash on the TV screen, and this is a check to ensure that your name is spelled correctly.

- Tip 5. Some interviewers, particularly when they are unprepared on a topic, will ask a question that seems "off the wall." This can also occur on a TV panel when another speaker veers off the topic or during an audience question and answer period. As in a radio interview, you must be prepared to use bridge phrases to return to the topic at hand.

- Tip 6. You can get media practice by listening and watching media interviews. Notice that even during a "hot" but good interview, the person being interviewed will tell his or her rendition of the event and not directly respond to the reporter's questions, particularly if these questions are accusatory or antagonistic. Truly professional interviewees will maintain their cool and stick to their points. For example, when a corporate executive of a company that has just polluted a river is being interviewed on the news, notice how he or she will describe the event and not be derailed by the reporter's attitude. The representative stays composed and sticks to the point, the object being to preserve the reputation of the company and explain "the company's side" of the story. Watching these pressure interviews can help you prepare for a difficult media experience.
- Tip 7. Any well-stocked bookstore will have books on working with the media, and many psychotherapy organizations offer literature and media training as part of their services. One example is a free booklet *How to Work with the Media: Interview Preparation for the Psychologist*. As an alternative, expert media coaches are available to teach you specific skills. Often they will videotape your presentation and review it with you. Both booklet and media training contacts are provided in the resource section at the end of this book.
- Tip 8. Karen Kalish (1999) suggests that when sitting during a TV interview, you lean slightly forward in the chair and remember that the microphone may be on. As a final sendoff, Karen says, "Look at every interview as a glorious opportunity. Smile."

HOW TO GET INTERVIEWED IN THE PRINT MEDIA AND ON RADIO AND TELEVISION

Print Media

Local smaller newspapers will often welcome articles on a variety of issues that are current for the month or season. For example, submit an article or information to the editor about holiday blues in November or separation issues with children beginning school in August. Larger city newspapers usually are staffed by many journalists, full time and part-time, who write lifestyle stories. It may be trickier to make connections with one or a couple of these reporters, but do not let that stop you. You can send some fact sheets, brochures, or pitch letters pertaining to a specific issue. You can send it to all the reporters who usually cover the kinds of stories that are related to your expertise or to psychological issues in general. Use the web site of the newspaper for faster and easier communication with several journalists at once.

Another means of getting interviewed and quoted may be to follow a story that has ongoing articles. If you have a psychological issue that pertains to the story, you can call it into the reporter. For example, major disasters are usually covered for several days. Send some points of information helpful to the readers, the survivors, and so on to the reporters who are carrying the story. When you make contact with the journalists, mention that you are available as needed on a variety of psychological issues. Be certain that they have your name and all the information they need to contact you. Then, periodically contact the person. From time to time send more information, another pitch letter or fact sheet. Be available again at the next disaster.

Radio

You have a good chance of getting on radio and a far greater chance of being heard on radio. When a news event that is related to your specialty occurs, you can call the newsroom with a comment. You may immediately be tape recorded and then your information may be repeated on the air during the next newscast. Therefore, if you do decide to call the newsroom, do all your preparing first. Go over all the radio points listed earlier in this section. Write down your three points. Be prepared for a question and answer time or, more likely, after getting your permission to be taped, they will tell you to just start talking. Make your points and be sure they have your name and location of your practice; that's all there is to it. In a later broadcast you may hear the reporter paraphrase your comments. He or she may give you credit if you are offering the information; sometimes they will include that you are a local psychotherapist or name the town or city. If they actually use some of your taped comments they will surely give you credit. Typically, your comments will be reduced to 15 seconds.

After you have made contact with a news reporter, be sure that he or she has your name and information correctly. Inform the reporter that you are willing to be called for further information either on this topic or on other future topics. If you are willing, you may tell the reporter that you can be available 24 hours a day if there is an urgent situation in which they would want a psychological point of view.

Television

It is often easier to create your own show on local access television than most people think. Local access stations are often looking for programs to schedule. They run 24 hours a day and frequently request a 30-minute segment that they will repeat at various hours around the clock for about 2 weeks. Every local access station has its own rules, requirements, and charges. Some have a nominal fee for taping and use of their studio. The programming is usually concerned with community education. A talk on marriage, divorce, step-parenting, and so on may be of interest to the station manager.

Where to start?

- Tip 1. Call your local access station and discuss the requirements with the station manager. You may be surprised to learn how easy this can be. Once you have some good tapes of programs you do, you have a product to help sell yourself to larger stations.
- Tip 2. Become familiar with the stations in your area. What stations have programming that could include you, a talk show that includes "expert" professionals, and so on. Of course, be cautious about entering an entertainment environment instead of one that will appreciate and respect you professionally.

Media interviews are not for everyone. They can be emotionally draining and time consuming. Media expert and psychologist Steve Brody[1] gives voice to this concern: "The media can be more of a drain than a practice builder if your energy and enthusiasm are channeled away from your clients, and your media or marketing work doesn't link or transfer well to your practice. . . . Media work, albeit exciting and romantic, can hurt rather than help a practice if you get too carried away with it."

On the other hand, psychologist Lenore Walker[2] notes that "TV work gets your message out to the public very quickly and efficiently. It usually gets lots of recognition and often leads to other media contacts if it is a national audience. This is a real positive for me."

Irene Deitch,[3] a psychologist who has been active in television and hosts her own cable TV show, says "Doing media is tough . . . your best shot becoming a 'media maven' is cable television. It allows for the greatest freedom and subject diversity. . . . The more you do it, the better you get, the more confident you will feel and the more you undertake."

With a caveat of caution, we present the upside and the downside to media interviews and suggest that you give it a try and learn what works for you and your practice.

NOTES

[1] Personal communication, June 3, 1999.
[2] Personal communication, April 16, 1999.
[3] Personal communication, May 12, 1999.

REFERENCES

American Psychological Association. (1999). How to work with the media: Interview preparation for the psychologist. New York: Office of Public Relations, APA.

Kalish, K. (1999). Press Kit. Washington, DC: Kalish Communications.

Chapter 17

Advanced Web Sites, Virtual Groups, Online Counseling, E-zines, and Electronic Publishing

It is predicted that Internet technology may have a societal impact that equals or exceeds that of the industrial revolution. This technological phenomenon, whose traffic doubles every hundred days, has enabled every individual to enter a world where a click on a computer mouse provides an instant opportunity for new information or a new connection (Jerome, 2000). Of relevance to psychotherapists is the creation of a consumer-based management of both health-related and mental health problems through online services. This new format of sharing health-related information through technology is known as telehealth and refers to services that combine telecommunication and health-related information. The use of online services for mental health issues is also referred to as psychotechnology. Telehealth connections offer many professional possibilities, including assessment and diagnosis, education, and consultation with clients on mental health issues. In addition, real time video cameras may be added to computers and telephones, enhancing these telecommunications.

As mental health professionals enter cyberspace, their professional world changes by expanding both the definition and the scope of their psychotherapeutic work. Psychotherapists in cyberspace can deliver unique psychological services from an office without walls. When such services are carefully and selectively offered to clients, the Internet offers a format for delivery of services that can be efficient, convenient, and effective.

ADVANCED WEB SITE

An advanced Web site is your virtual office, and its appearance and function are analogous to your physical office. How you use color, pictures, literature, magazines, and music determines the nature and feeling of your virtual setting. New and current clients can enter your virtual office at any time and find out your specialization, location, and credentials. They do not need you to be physically present to hear you giving a presentation, watch a short video about you and your work, or buy some of the items you sell. Clients can go to your chat room, communicate through e-mail, or find out about your e-groups or e-counseling sessions. You can feature your current workshops or a professional section about supervision and courses. Your virtual office home page can have moving graphics, links to other sites, and a question and answer section.

Example of an Advanced Web Site

There are a number of features that make the Web site shown in Figure 17.1 distinctive. A series of buttons on the left side of the home page serve as an index and take the reader to a specific feature. The first few buttons offer a brief biography of the therapist and a series of articles in the therapist's specialty area, designed to demonstrate competency and stimulate interest. The fourth button displays information about telephone self-esteem workshops (virtual groups described later). A separate question and answer button permits the reader to interact with the therapist through e-mailed conversation. Following this is a page that provides a comprehensive description, editorial review, and ordering information about books the Web site owner has edited or coauthored. The final button provides a link to other psychotherapists in different geographic areas with a variety of different specialties.

Note that in the center of the home page is a button for "video clips." Excerpts of television interviews provide examples of the psychotherapist's interview and speaking ability, a useful feature for the media and those looking to hire a public speaker. Finally, a "What's New" button provides recent, reader-friendly information on applied psychology.

VIRTUAL GROUPS: COMPUTER BASED

A virtual group is a group of individuals who join together for a specific purpose but do not need to occupy the same space. There are many differences between types of online groups. They can be scheduled

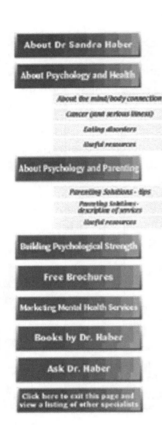

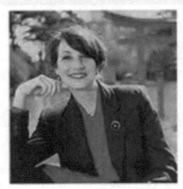

Dr. Sandra Haber

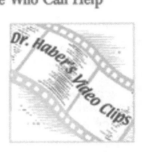

Talk To Someone Who Can Help

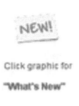

Click graphic for

"What's New"

Click graphic for

"VideoClips" page

Her newest book, *Saying Good-Bye to Managed Care: Building Your Independent Psychotherapy Practice,* will soon be available (Springer Publishing).

* About Dr. Sandra Haber
* About the Mind/Body connection
* Cancer (and Serious Illness): Alternative Medicine and Psychology
* About Psychology and Parenting: Parenting Solution Tips
* Building Psychological Strength Through Self-Esteem
* ask Dr Haber (send e-mail questions)
* Books by Dr. Haber
* Click here to exit this page and view a listing of other specialists

FIGURE 17.1 Example of an advanced Web site.

and structured or informal, intermittent, and loosely structured. Concrete and emotional issues are discussed in online groups. There are traditional and nontraditional forums with peers or professional facilitators, or both.

In professional online groups, e-mail can be used for the initial screening and history of the group member. Usually the real name of the client and other intake information are noted, as well as the screen name. After clients are assessed and accepted, they are placed into a group according to their needs, just as in real groups.

Online chat rooms are an example of a virtual group in which members write in and communicate with other members on a specific topic of mutual interest. Some mental health professionals and several health-related organizations have begun to use this format for people with similar problems. In these cases, many of these groups are led by professional therapists. Clinicians can be invited to be guest speakers at one of these groups, depending on areas of expertise. It is important to note that a number of electronic health services (telehealth services primarily driven by economics rather than professional education) offer chat rooms that are not professionally led.

Advantages

- Connects individuals who live in different geographic areas and individuals who are convalescing, housebound, or disabled with an expert, and they can share experiences with other individuals in similar situations.
- Connects people with special needs for support and resource information.
- Increases professional visibility.
- The psychotherapist-researcher finds that virtual groups rooms can yield a wealth of data and clinical vignettes.
- Professional group leaders are frequently paid for online time.

Disadvantages

- This is a text-based environment, and there is a need for the participants to be literate, have the ability to express feelings in words, be honest, and type clearly.
- Interpersonal and visual cues from the group are not available, and interactions are limited and time delayed by the system.
- Silence and not posting is perceived as absence.
- Guest experts leading chat room discussions are usually not reimbursed.

VIRTUAL GROUPS: TELEPHONE BASED

Another form of a virtual group uses the telephone. As with a computer group, a virtual telephone group can be "advertised" on your advanced Web site, although the actual service is delivered by telephone. Participants of the group will need to be screened in advance of the group to determine their suitability to this format. This most closely resembles a conference call. The psychotherapist expert then leads a telephone workshop on a specific topic or for a series of telephone group sessions. Similar to group therapy, there is typically a fee for service, a structure to the meeting and the interaction, and a beginning, middle, and end to the session. In this situation, a group is given the number of a "bridge line" that they can use at a specific hour, at a specified period of time (see Appendix).

Advantages

- Verbal cues, voice intonation, and content of communication are available to the therapist and group participants.
- Participants can call in from anywhere in the world as long as they have access to a telephone.
- Participants can maintain anonymity by using simply their first name or pseudonym, particularly useful for shy or easily recognized individuals.
- Modality is particularly helpful for individuals with restricted mobility, whether it is due to physical impairment, geographic residence or other limiting condition.
- The therapist increases the likelihood of forming a group because geography is a nonissue.
- The number of participants is limited only by the size of the group the therapist can run (as opposed to the size of a professional office).
- Fees depend on the number and length of the sessions.

Disadvantages

- The therapist needs to be able to have sufficient enrollment to have a group process and to make the group practical financially.
- The therapist must arrange payment by establishing a credit card acceptance or by receiving checks by mail, or both.
- The therapist must rent a bridge line, which is different than an operated assisted telephone conference call. A bridge line is less expensive than a conference call is. Suppliers of bridge and teleconferencing lines are listed in the Appendix.

- A strong, content-focused session must be developed for a workshop.
- One difficult or inappropriate caller can cause havoc in a virtual telephone group.

Example of a Virtual Group

One of the authors (SH) offered a virtual workshop in building self-esteem. She wrote up flyers and distributed them to her current patients; mailed them to her old patients, whom she thought might be interested; and contacted colleagues for referral possibilities, to whom she sent flyers. She also invited a guest, owner of a local fitness program, to be in on the call at no charge to ascertain if the content would be appropriate for her clients in the future.

Group members prepaid for the workshop by check or credit card. Registrants were contacted the day before the workshop and given a call-in phone number. The day of the workshop, all registrants called the number at a specific time. An 11-person connection was established, and a virtual group on self-esteem skills was run. In this case, because most of the participants were local, the leader rented a teleconferencing line and paid the charges. If the group were more national, it would have been financially prudent to rent a long distance bridge line and have each member pay his or her own charges.

A formal training program in telephone coaching is offered by Ben Dean (1999). His MentorCoach program provides training in niche market carve out and Web-based newsletters and in setting up and running virtual telephone groups. "Coaching is a natural option for therapists interested in diversification outside of Managed Care. It's an exploding new profession and we have every right to be part of it" (Dean, 2000).

ONLINE COUNSELING

Online therapy counseling services have jumped from 12 in 1996 to 162 in 1999 and are becoming a more acknowledged option for providing psychoeducational services (Gormley, 1999). Online therapy uses e-mail, instant messages, or one of the online therapy services, or a combination of these, for individual client "sessions."

According to *Psychotherapy Finances* (1999) there is a range of online therapists who use this form of communication from a "steady sideline to a practice staple." Some are committed to building a "distant" therapy practice with telephone and e-mail "advice"; others are working on developing a " library of stock answers" to common problems that can be adapted and personalized.

Psychotherapy online is unregulated. A cybertherapist does not have to have any credentials. As of this writing, the federal government has yet to pass laws governing online counseling, permitting each state to define and manage the practice themselves. The major psychotherapy organizations have also not yet adopted a clear policy about this form of service delivery. There are, however, two online verification sites that have established a credentialing system. You can join and be cited in the directory of Internet psychotherapists; several are listed in the Appendix of this book.

Potential problems of online psychotherapy include:

- an inability to see the patient and discern important physical cues
- a difficulty determining the identity of patient
- miscommunication either from therapist to patient or from patient to therapist
- potential breaches in confidentiality
- lack of knowledge of legal requirements and community resources in the client's hometown

In an Internet review of online psychotherapy, it was noted that

The American Psychological Association supports and encourages the ethical use of tele-health . . . However, there is not yet a good body of research on the topic; psychologists are still pulling out what does and doesn't work. Email is fine for exchanging information, but seems to break down where it becomes necessary to make decisions around contentious issues. (Brauner, 1999)

Diana List Cullen (1995), social worker–psychotherapist, shares some of her thoughts about online work:

One of my primary principles is to treat every inquiry or comment as if the person were presenting an actual problem and situation. I decided early on that I would rather risk someone having a good laugh at putting one over on the therapist than risk disbelieving a legitimate story and concern. I also thought that if someone were making up a story, it was likely to be a metaphor . . . ."

A recent Web site, Here2Listen, sanctioned by experts from leading medical schools and university psychology departments, has taken a more aggressive approach in validating online counseling. In a company press release, the owners of the site note that online counseling offers a practical way for therapists and counselors to expand their services and simplify their practice . . . (the service) will enable therapists and counselors to meet new clients, conduct counseling sessions, manage their billing and scheduling, access hundreds of industry resources, chat with peers, achieve credential verification and connect with insurance providers . . . (counseling) will create a new forum for therapists to help patients who may be unable to travel to an office, uncomfortable with traditional therapy or in need of immediate help.

E-ZINES AND E-NEWSLETTERS

An e-zine is an online magazine that can have text articles, photos, graphics, audio, and video clips. Anything that can be done on the Web can be done on an e-zine. Generally, a consumer or client subscribes to an e-zine. E-zines are easy to read because the consumer receives only the front page and an index and then chooses items of interest. If you wish to publish and e-mail your own e-zine, there are sites that will help you do this.

An online newsletter is usually not as complex as an e-zine and is generally more text oriented. The client or consumer can subscribe to an e-newsletter.

In his article on writing a reader-friendly e-mail newsletter, psychologist Ben Dean (1999) recommends that you learn formatting techniques and e-mail writing skills. He suggests the following:

- your e-mail newsletter should begin with a wisely selected target market
- a single idea, concisely treated, is enough
- write in plain text
- use narrow line widths
- use "hard carriage returns"
- understand the importance of the subject line
- be succinct and concise
- write for scannability

Example of an E-Newsletter

Ron Fox and Mike Thomas operate a Web site aimed at individuals in family businesses. Free monthly newsletters are e-mailed to anyone who is interested. The current issue and back issues are available on their Web site (www.FamilyBusinessdoctor.com). Each newsletter is focused on a different substantive aspect of family business. Examples include "Three Keys to a Successful Family Business," "Family Business Retreats," and "How to Retain High Performance Employees." Fox notes that

> People can subscribe or unsubscribe to my free monthly electronic newsletter with very little trouble. They also can read and print past issues. The newsletter is my primary method for opening communication with potential clients and it reaches them wherever they may be located! Although my subscriber base is still small, I already have subscribers from some European and Pacific Basin countries.

VIRTUAL PUBLISHING

Virtual publishing is an alternative for the psychotherapist who wants to publish a book, be it professional or trade. According to recent statistics, more than 50% of the sales in the electronic book category are professional books with an average price of $3.47 per book (Carvajal, 2000). Although a maverick idea at its inception, virtual publishing has begun to capture the attention of traditional publishing houses who often post excerpts of coming books in the virtual stores. To evaluate whether virtual publishing is right for you, first clarify your goals. Are you trying to establish your credibility and reputation? Are you trying to make money? Do you want to reach a wide audience? Russell Galen, in an interview with D. Carvajal,

> If I had a young author whose career I was trying to build I'd rather have a hundred dollars from The New Yorker than a thousand from Fatbrain. But with my 82-year-old author my concern is reaching readers. He doesn't need money. He doesn't need prestige. He just wants to change lives.

Examples of virtual publishing sites include Fatbrain, 1stbooks, and 1universe. Details are listed in the Appendix.

FINAL WORDS ABOUT AN ADVANCED WEB SITE

In the words of Web-site owner–psychologist Ron Fox,[1] "Web sites can be a way to market and sell services and products to audiences anywhere in the world. That is a mind-boggling opportunity. But it will not come knocking on your door. You must go after it."

NOTE

[1] Personal communication, January 7, 2000.

REFERENCES

Brauner, A-M. (1999, June 10). Cybertherapy: Ready for prime time? [On-Line]. WebMD

Carvajal, D. (2000, February 7). Virtual publishing: From Arthur Clarke to psoriasis tales. *The New York Times*, p. 1.

Cullen, D. L. (1995, Summer). Psychotherapy in cyberspace. *Clinician, 26,* 3.

Dean, B. (1999, Fall). Building a coaching or consulting practice: Writing a reader-friendly email newsletter. *Independent Practitioner,* 105–109.

Dean B. (2000, February 28). [www.MentorCoach.com]

Fox, R., & Thomas, M. [www.FamilyBusinessDoctor.com]

Gormley, B. (1999, June 6). Online counseling service growing. *Providence Business News,* 1.

Here2Listen.com Launches eCounseling Web Site. (2000, January 20). Press release.

Jerome, L. (2000, February 25). Presentation to Council of the American Psychological Association.

Will on line "therapy" become standard practice? (1999, September). *Psychotherapy Finances,* pp. 9–10.

Chapter 18

Advertising

Advertising is an added expense, so it needs to be seriously considered before being added as a marketing tool. The sine qua non of advertising is repetition, and therefore it is a long-term endeavor. If you can sustain an ongoing advertising budget, if you choose your advertising vehicle wisely, and if you create an interesting and appealing ad, then advertising may be an important aspect of practice building. Of all the public relations possibilities, paid-for advertising remains the one to be approached most thoughtfully.

In general, we suggest that mental health practitioners consider four relatively affordable forms of advertising: Yellow Page ads, ads in hometown and specialty newspapers, targeted mailings, and barter offsets. Other forms of advertising, such as direct mail, national magazines, and radio and television, are generally too costly for the average practitioner to sustain over time, and a one-time exposure, although more financially viable, is usually not considered to be a worthwhile approach.

YELLOW PAGE ADS

Yellow page ads can usually be purchased for a reasonable amount of money. These ads are appealing because the consumer is actively searching for a product or a service.

In deciding whether or not to advertise in the Yellow Pages, consider what follows.

Information Gathering

Almost all psychotherapists are listed in the "yellow pages" of at least one directory. These basic listings are "free" and are part of your business line advantage. Once you add to the basic, fees increase and decisions need to be made. You have choices of having your name and phone number in bold type, adding a line to the usual two-line listing, or having a 1/2 inch listing. Then you may choose a boxed ad of increasing size and you can add color (usually red or blue). Talk with your local phone company for the pricing on all these options to learn exactly what the incremental costs will be.

In deciding on whether to purchase a more expensive ad, try to ascertain how successful other psychotherapists have been through this type of advertising. The experience of colleagues can provide valuable data about what works and what does not work. Not everyone will be willing to share their results, but it is worth a try.

Another way of ascertaining success is to obtain an older Yellow Pages book and see if the same individuals have advertised before, or ask the sales representative if specific individuals will appear in the next edition. If their Yellow Page ad was a success, you will see them advertising again and again.

Decision Making

Once you have gathered your information about costs and professional experiences, you will still have to make a decision. Should you or should you not spend this extra money? On the one hand, in a service profession, people usually prefer a word of mouth referral. The Yellow Pages will only appeal to those who do not have such a network or are too hesitant to reveal their need. However, there can be large numbers of people in this last category. From what we have learned a Yellow Page ad does pay off with increased referrals if you have either a specific specialty or your ad is unique. Do you have the time, energy, and possibly financing to make your ad outstanding?

Creating an Outstanding Ad

Look at the ads that are already listed. Your ad will need to be "bigger or better" than the others. This can be accomplished by being bigger, more colorful, or more appealing. According to *Psychotherapy Finances* (1999), which reviewed Yellow Page ads coast to coast, sometimes ads work and sometimes they do not: ". . . eschewing the traditional black and white listings, many clinicians are creating large display ads with multi-color layouts, personal photos, and eye-grabbing headlines . . . the overall trend indicates that therapists are experimenting in an effort to garner a larger share of the market. . . ."

Although, better and bigger are self-explanatory and relevant for product advertising, these factors may well be less relevant in advertising a personal service. "Appealing" may well be more important than either bigger or better when it comes to a personal service.

Design an ad that has a personal feeling to it, remembering that you are offering a personal, intimate service. Notice in Figure 18.1 Joyce Sachs has a very appealing design and a very appealing message.

To have an ad similar to that of Joyce Sachs you will need to work with a designer and send the telephone company camera-ready copy. For line space, even up to several inches, where no design is necessary, the phone company will usually help you to lay it out at no extra charge. Joyce Sachs[1] has such an outstanding ad that she reports getting many patients each year from the Yellow Pages.

Another successful approach may come from multiple listings. For example, a person who has a weight problem might look under psychotherapist, weight control, or counseling, or all of these. A parent of a child with ADHD might look under psychotherapist, learning, tutors, or education, or all of these. A well-designed ad that appears in each location will have the repetition factor, creating an advantage. Remember that most of the public identifies with the specific problem; they do not necessarily associate psychological help or psychotherapy with a solution to their problem.

Above all, in creating an outstanding ad, remember to answer the question: what makes your service special? If you have a specific specialty (marital problems, ADHD), an appealing location (on Main Street), convenient hours of business (Saturday appointments), manageable fees (accept insurance or sliding scale), or other special features, be sure that this information appears prominently in your ad.

COMMUNITY AND HOMETOWN NEWSPAPERS

Community and hometown newspapers are worthy considerations for your advertising dollars. Marketing expert Kim Ricketts[2] notes that community papers are well read. "Statistics show that people tend to read their community papers cover to cover versus 'scanning' the larger papers."

Some communities have general community newspapers as well as smaller specialty newspapers. For example, in one community there may be a paper on parenting, another on senior activities, and another on sports events. All are distributed free of charge. There are also numerous flyer types of newspapers: from the local health club, yoga center, gay and lesbian club, and so on. All of these printed materials

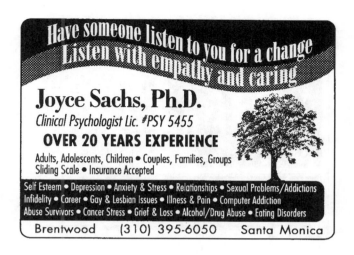

FIGURE 18.1   Yellow pages ad.

tend to be read by a specific targeted audience and are places to consider advertising.

Stacy Steingart[3] of Big Apple Parents, emphasizes the importance of the targeted audience. She makes an analogy to the traditional real estate advice of "location! location! location!" and suggests that the same thinking applies to psychotherapy advertising. "An in-the-face, yet gentle approach is best. Choose your target, place your ads, and get ready for the amazing results."

Cheryl Perlman (2000), a clinical social worker who specializes in eating disorders, placed a small ad in a local paper and local magazine (Figure 18.2). She noted that the ad was very successful but responses only came in after a few months. In advertising, the general advice is repetition, repetition, repetition. Once you select a publication, prepare to make a reasonable time commitment (about 6 months) before you evaluate the results.

Local newspaper ads cost far less than do ads in larger newspapers and, in fact, are more desirable. Local advertising tends to focus on clients who are familiar with the location of your office and can get there easily. Local newspapers frequently give special prices for purchase of a series of ads. Call your local newspaper for quotes on their pricing.

If you do advertise in a local paper, consider sending a pitch letter to the editor (see chapter 15) so that a news story can also appear in the paper. For example, if your ad is about psychotherapy to help

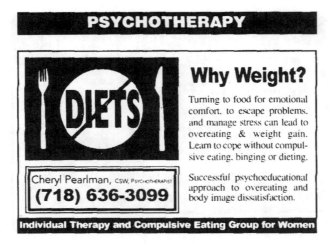

FIGURE 18.2   Community newspaper ad.

people lose weight, it would be helpful to pitch an article about the "Psychology of Weight Loss: How People can Stay Motivated on a Diet." An interview mentioning your name will bolster your advertising message by adding a credibility factor to your work.

POSTCARDS

Some therapists have begun to use postcards in a targeted mailing campaign as an advertising strategy for a specific part of their practice.

Rosemary Lavinski, social worker–psychotherapist uses a post card to advertise her web site and get others involved in her groups. Her card has an interesting design and is a followup on her brochure and stationery (Figure 18.3).

Another clever use of a postcard was by Dolores Walker and Carol Butler (Figure 18.4). They used this format to advertise their book and work in divorce mediation. It is easy to read and remember and even easier to find out about their work.

For this type of advertising, there are costs of graphic layout, postcard production, and mailing costs. If your mailing list is very focused and has an audience that is interested in your services, it may be a cost that is worth pursuing.

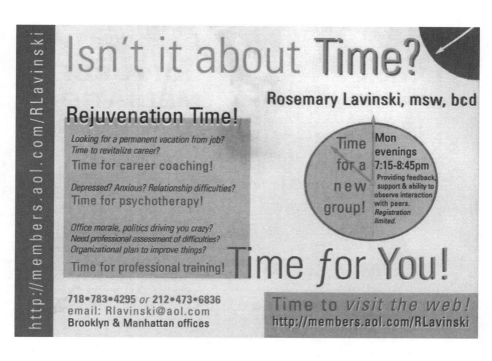

FIGURE 18.3 Postcard.

BARTER OFFSET

An interesting arrangement that can be relatively low cost is "barter off-set." In this case, a small advertising medium exchanges advertising space for your service. For example, when Ellen McGrath,[4] psychologist-author and well-known speaker, was asked to deliver a keynote address at a state psychology association, she learned that they could only pay a portion of her speaking fee. She agreed to do the speech, but asked for free advertising for her book in the next few issues of their newsletter.

Similarly, in chapter 13 we discussed holding a workshop on the premises of a small business. Small business often have ongoing ads, and most would be happy to feature your name in exchange for a workshop held on site.

Another type of barter offset is advertising in a nonprofit fund-raising event. In this case, you pay for advertising but the costs are often tax deductible. You get the benefit of being known as a supporter of a worthwhile charity and event, as well as the chance to advertise your services or product to a like-minded audience.

Save time, money and emotional energy with a mediated separation or divorce

The Divorce Mediation Answer Book
By Carol A. Butler, Ph.D and
Dolores D. Walker, C.S.W., J.D.

"Amidst the plethora of divorce mediation material now available, this book by psychotherapist Butler and attorney Walker helps simplify the issues." —*Library Journal*

"Here is an 'answer' book that I would highly recommend to both mediators and clients." —*Academy of Family Mediators*

"I highly recommend this helpful and informative guide." —*Dan Couvrette, Publisher, Divorce Magazine*

Available at local bookstores or by calling (800) 451-7556
ISBN -56836-262-8 $16.00

Kodansha, 575 Lexington Ave., NY, NY 10022
Publicity Manager: Nicki Britton (917) 322-6236
For publicity please contact:

Questions about mediation? I'm on the 11th fl.
Dolores Walker, CSW, JD (212) 691-6073

The

DIVORCE MEDIATION ANSWER BOOK

SAVE TIME, MONEY, AND EMOTIONAL ENERGY WITH A MEDIATED SEPARATION OR DIVORCE

Carol A. Butler, Ph.D., and
Dolores D. Walker, M.S.W., JD.

FIGURE 18.4   Answer book.

In conclusion, advertising will usually cost you money. In the long run, you must assess whether your return on your investment will make your advertising worth it. A grandiose plan can be very costly; a timid plan can be a wasted effort. Assess your practice, and your needs and review your options. Remember, advertising is just one part of marketing and usually the final tool to be added.

NOTES

[1] Personal communication, April 23, 1999.
[2] Personal communication, March 3, 1999.
[3] Personal communication, January 12, 1999.
[4] Personal communication, June 1, 1999.

REFERENCES

American Psychological Association. (1998). How to work with the media: Interview preparation for the psychologist. New York: Office of Public Relations, APA.

Trends: Coast to coast, therapists are getting bolder in the Yellow Pages. (1999). *Psychotherapy Finances, 25,* 1.

Part VII

Putting It All Together

Chapter 19

The Final Step to Success: Using What You Know to Create Your Independent Psychotherapy Practice

This chapter concludes our book and starts you on your path to a successful, independent psychotherapy practice. In the following pages, we demonstrate how to summarize and integrate your skills and marketing tools with a variety of marketable niche topics. We have divided this chapter into several sections. Each section will give you readily useable information and ways to implement the ideas presented.

PSYCHOTHERAPISTS AND RELATIONSHIPS: A NATURAL MARKETING EXAMPLE

Love makes the world go round. Love relationships and love experiences, be they fulfilled, spurned, lost or unrequited, are a topic of universal interest. Psychotherapists are experts in treating relationship issues. We are the gurus of relationships in all of their forms. We are the specialists who know about a range of intimate relationships as well as multifaceted family relationships. Every practicing therapist has dealt with some aspect of a relationship, and so it is a natural topic on which you can use your existing skills to create a specialty or niche market for your business.

In the next section, we have used the partnering cycle to provide two ready-to-use examples of niche marketing. For this, or any niche topic, the formula for success will be the same:

Gold Standard Skills + Long Term Marketing = Business Success

As you read through the many different faces of the relationship niche and begin to carve out your own specialty area, keep this formula in mind.

RELATIONSHIPS: A READY-TO-USE MARKETING NICHE

Example 1: Separation and Divorce

Is This a Marketable Niche?

A tried and true standby for most psychotherapy practices is taking on patients who anticipate, worry about, or are recovering from the process of separation and divorce.

Americans say that a happy marriage is their number one goal and 85 to 90% of our citizens continue to get married. Unfortunately, despite this goal, the divorce rate has remained the same for the past 30 years and is predicted to remain the same in the near future (Coalition for Marriage Family and Couples Education, 2000). Couples researcher John Gottmann reports that "more than half of all first marriages end in divorce. Second marriages do worse, failing at a rate of about 60 percent" (1994, p. 16).

These figures speak to a huge population of potential patients who are in serious need of psychological help. We know that marital distress causes increased risk for mental and physical problems in adults and children and that conflicts in the home lead to decreased productivity in the work environment.

For many, the process of separation and divorce activates deep feelings of failure, loss, abandonment, and guilt. Psychotherapists traditionally help individuals and couples deal with issues around communication, money, children, and their future. Psychotherapy can be valuable for managing the immediate crisis as well as for fostering the changes that would be instrumental in increasing the likelihood of success in a future marriage.

Fortunately, the public is open to psychotherapists helping with relationship concerns. In a study by the APA (1996), 29% of those asked said that they would be "very likely to consult" a mental health professional for divorce or marital problems and 62% said they would be "very/somewhat likely to consult" a mental health professional for this problem.

Achieving the Gold Standard of Skills

If you decide to use the topic of separation and divorce as a niche market, begin by giving yourself several months to assess and develop your current professional skills Consider your current practice and those of your colleagues. Take a good look at what you know and what you will need to know to become an expert. Be sure to consider your education, supervision, and experience. Find out what other experts do in this area and how successful they are. To improve on your existing skills, consider attending workshops and conferences offered by your national, state, or local professional association. Checking out continuing education classes as well as supervisors who are expert in this area can quickly bring you up to speed. Consider online courses and reading the latest journal research and books written by respected researchers in the field of relationships, couples, marriage, and divorce. If you need to further your clinical experience, consider volunteering your services at a local hospital, mental health clinic, or public service facility.

Shaping Your Marketing Materials

As you sharpen your skills, you will refine your target population and begin to conceptualize the marketing approach you will take. Do you need additional stationery or business cards that highlight your niche area? Can you devise talks or workshops that provide a "hook" or angle for the topic of separation and divorce? Begin to formulate your workshop, community talk, or community newspaper article with this packaging in mind. The following are samples of marketing materials that are angled for the separation and divorce niche.

The press release for a hometown paper shown in Figure 19.1 features a workshop that addresses a prevalent concern of separated and divorced parents. Notice the bookstore setting, a natural arena in which to feature this talk.

Another marketing tool focused on the separation and divorce niche features a virtual telephone group for single parents of teenagers. We know that two-parent households with teenage children feel overwhelmed and we know that single parents feel overwhelmed, so it is reasonable to assume that single parents of teenagers suffer a double whammy of stress. A virtual telephone group offers the presence and support of others in a similar life situation and has the added feature of enabling the overwhelmed parent to participate from home. To shape your virtual group you will need a plan that addresses the following issues:

- Is this a one-time event or series of telephone sessions?
- Will there be a fee? If yes, what will it be?
- If you are charging a fee, how will you collect it? Will fees be paid in advance or after services are rendered?

FOR IMMEDIATE RELEASE   MAY 5, 2000

                                                        Contact: Frank Brown, Ph.D.

                                                        212-123-4567

DIVORCE: WHAT DO WE TELL THE CHILDREN?

Half of all marriages end in divorce, and many of these include families with children. A common worry is what to tell the children. On Wednesday, June 1, psychotherapist Frank Brown will present a workshop on "Divorce: What Do We Tell The Children." The workshop will be held in Community Bookstore, at 456 Ocean Street at 7:30 PM.

Most parents who are contemplating divorce are in a quandary when it comes to their children. When should you tell a child about a separation or divorce? How should you tell them? If the separation or divorce involves an extra-marital affair, should this be disclosed? How can each parent maintain an active loving relationship with their children while the family is dissolving?

These, and other questions, will be addressed by psychotherapist Brown.

Following this talk, tip sheets will be distributed and a sample of helpful books, courtesy of Community Bookstore will be on display. A questions and answer period will follow the workshop. The workshop is free, but registration is required. To register, call 212-123-4567 before May 22.

FIGURE 19.1   Press release.

- Do you want to take credit cards? See the Appendix for information about the Visa credit card.
- Write down a structured content for each session. What will your participants learn from this session? Will you teach any techniques or give any "homework"?
- Write down a series of open-ended questions that you can use throughout the phone call to encourage discussion and group participation.
- Make the arrangements for renting a bridge line so that you can offer this call at the lowest possible cost (see Appendix).
- How will you recruit your participants? Develop a flyer and a networking list of professional and personal contacts.

A brochure is another useful tool. Figure 19.2 is an example of a ready-made brochure that you can purchase and have personally imprinted. See the Appendix for ordering information.

Web sites and e-zines are effective ways to establish a continuing dialogue with potential clientele. Divorce and separation information can appear as a separate section within your own Web site, as a feature on someone else's Web site, or as a Web site entity in and of itself (see for example, smartmarriages.com). In all cases, you will need to have information appearing on a regular basis that will be of interest to your audience. Some topics related to the niche of separation and divorce are

- going to events as a single
- getting through the holidays when you are newly divorced or separated
- fun things to do with your children
- dating again: 10 tips of returning to the singles scene
- learning from a failed marriage
- being a single parent to a teenager

Each of the previous topics could be enlarged into a tip sheet or one-page information sheet and posted as part of a Web service or e-zine.

Developing Your Networking Contacts and Marketing Distribution Plan

Once you have refined your marketing products you need to determine how you will distribute them. The key to a successful marketing is contact with other professionals and the public. Since separation and divorce issues are major areas of patient concern, our colleagues are often looking for referral sources, particularly if they are doing individual therapy with one member of a couple that is in conflict. Typically, they will need an individual therapist for the other member of the couple or a couples therapist for the individuals together. Other needs include those of the individual children and the entire family. To obtain individual patient referrals, you can begin to network at professional meetings, over lunch, or in any of the various ways previously outlined.

Because you have already developed a workshop or community talk, you would also be networking with other community resources and offering your services. One ongoing marketing plan for your niche would be to use your workshop or community talk as a springboard for advertising other services, such as your virtual telephone group, Web site, and e-zine. Remember that a workshop or series of workshops on different aspects of separation and divorce has good value-added potential for hosting by churches and synagogues, bookstores, and community service groups such as the local YM/YWCA.

When a marriage ends everyone in the family hurts.

YOU OR YOUR CHILDREN MIGHT FEEL...

- Anxious
- Sad
- Angry
- Ashamed
- Confused
- Fearful
- Depressed
- Helpless
- Resentful
- Embarrassed
- Lonely
- Guilty

YOU OR YOUR CHILDREN MAY...

- Be more forgetful or irritable
- Have difficulty at work or school
- Struggle with eating, sleeping concentrating or cry more often
- Have fleeting thoughts of death or dying

All of these feelings, thoughts and behaviors are normal. You and your children may experience some or all of them.

ISSUES YOUR FAMILY WILL FACE...

- Telling your children, family and friends
- Negotiating a separation agreement
- A possible change in residence
- A possible change in school
- A possible change in financial status
- A new job or return to work
- Adjusting to your ex-spouse's new relationships

HOW TO HELP YOURSELF

- STAY CONNECTED TO OTHERS
  Spend time with friends and family.
- EXERCISE AND EAT RIGHT
  These are two of the best ways to cope.
- KEEP A JOURNAL
  It's a great outlet for your feelings.
- CONSIDER A SUPPORT GROUP
  Sharing your feelings can help.
- CONTACT A PSYCHOLOGIST
  Get help if you or your children experience prolonged difficulties.

TELLING YOUR CHILDREN

- Tell your children when the decision to separate is definite.
- Try to tell your children about the decision to divorce together using words they can understand.
- Assure your children of your love and that you will still be part of their lives.
- Be specific about the changes that will happen in their lives.

When their parents separate children feel that their world has fallen apart. The majority of children will recover and heal. Children can have the same feelings as adults. However, they differ in their understanding and control of feelings. On-going hostility and conflict between their parents can result in life-long problems for children.

"All they did was fight all the time. I could hear them late at night. They said really bad things to each other. I used to lie in my bed and cry all the time. Now they're going to get a divorce. I'm so scared."

CHILDREN OFTEN EXPRESS THEIR FEELINGS AND FANTASIES THROUGH THEIR BEHAVIOR

Your child may...

- Act out at home or school
- Have fluctuating or poor grades
- Be angry and uncooperative
- Cling and cry more easily
- Have trouble paying attention
- Appear uptight and tense
- Have trouble eating or sleeping
- Withdraw from family or friends
- Think they caused the divorce

HOW TO HELP YOUR CHILDREN

- BE EXTRA AFFECTIONATE
  This is a time when children need increased warmth and affection.
- MAINTAIN REGULAR STRUCTURE AND DISCIPLINE
  This makes children feel safe and secure.
- SUPPORT YOUR CHILDREN'S FRIENDSHIPS AND ACTIVITIES
  Children need to stay connected to their own lives.
- DON'T BAD MOUTH OR BLAME YOUR SPOUSE
  Children have two parents. They want to love and be loyal to both of you.
- DON'T ASK YOUR CHILDREN TO TAKE CARE OF YOU
  Your children need you to be their parent. Avoid using them as a friend or confidant.

Talk to Someone Who Can Help.

Talk to Someone Who Can Help...

Separation and Divorce...

"I was sure that our marriage would last forever. Now it's over and I don't know what to do. My children's lives are ruined. I can't eat or sleep. No one will ever want me."

PSYCHOLOGISTS ARE SPECIALLY TRAINED to help you and your children recover from the trauma of a separation and divorce. A psychologist can work with you and your children to help you get through this stressful time.

ADJUSTING TO YOUR "NEW" SINGLE LIFE CAN BE DIFFICULT.

A psychologist can help you with many of the issues you will face including...

- Single Parenting
- Time Management
- Socializing and Dating
- Relationships with "His" or "Her" Family
- Co-Parenting with your Ex-Spouse
- Mediating Conflicts with your Ex-Spouse

Talk to Someone Who Can Help.

Prepared By: Alice Rubenstein, Ed.D., Sirout Black, Ph.D., J.D. and James Cosse, Ph.D.

THE BROCHURE PROJECT
A Joint Venture of the Divisions
of Psychotherapy and Independent Practice
American Psychological Association
Co-Directors:
Alice Rubenstein, Ed.D. and Sandra Haber, Ph.D.
Publication Coordinators:
Abraham Wolf, Ph.D. and Peter Sheras, Ph.D.
© The Brochure Project, 1998
(602) 854-8909

Separation and Divorce are Traumatic for the Entire Family

You and your children will have good days and bad days. Pay attention to patterns of behavior. If problems persist, get help.

A PSYCHOLOGIST CAN HELP WITH...

- Prolonged feelings of anxiety or depression.
- Feeling overwhelmed and unable to gain control of your life.
- Difficulty eating or sleeping.
- Difficulty concentrating at work, school or home.
- Difficulty expressing or controlling your feelings.
- Increased use of alcohol or drugs to self-medicate.
- Physical reactions including headaches, stomach aches and pains.

A Psychologist Can Help You Get Back on Your Feet

FIGURE 19.2 Brochure.

181

You can announce various professional offerings through materials left in your office, sent to other therapist and professionals, and distributed at workshops, such as the one listed in Figure 19.1.

Building a relationship with the media will also support your overall marketing game plan. Media reports need to reflect the concerns and interests of their readers. Susan Faludi (1991) noted the inaccuracy in reporting and harm that the media can create toward women. Faludi referred to a report that misquoted and misinterpreted that research had found that if a woman was unmarried by age 40, she had the same chance of getting married as being killed by a terrorist. When you are aware of inaccuracies in reporting, it offers you, the expert, a window of opportunity to pitch an interesting story. For example, in addition to correctly presenting the data you could offer to discuss obstacles to commitment, the advantages of later marriages, or the benefits and liabilities of being a single parent. With so many headline newstories relating to marriage and divorce, you can pitch a variety of possible angles to your favorite media outlet.

Other media-related possibilities for marketing separation and divorce issues are to focus on holiday time and use the pitch of "how to survive the first holiday season separated or divorced." "How will you celebrate, with whom, where will the children be, how will you handle invitations from friends and relatives."

As your last step, you will move into action. You have your ideas, you have determined what you will do and how you will do it, and now you spring to action. You have honed your gold standard skills and have a marketing plan. Your various materials have been sent to your networking contacts. Congratulations! You have carved out a specialty within the divorce and separation niche.

Example 2: The Wedding Niche

Is This a Marketable Niche?

Whereas separation and divorce is a crisis that most therapists work with, a more unusual spin on the relationship niche focuses on the beginning of a marital partnership. Several years ago, while shopping for a bridal gown, one of the authors (ER) began chatting with the shop owner regarding the horrors of mothers of the brides and how difficult they often make it for their daughters. So frequently, mothers behave as if the wedding were their own, creating pressures, anxieties, and resentments in both the bride and the groom. Having dealt with this issue professionally both with patients (brides) who were getting married and with their mothers it was very clear how a psychotherapist could be helpful in setting the stage for a more harmonious couple and in-law relationships in the future.

Achieving the Gold Standard of Skills

In this particular case, the psychotherapist already had the skills needed to be expert in this area, because her training and practice focused on couples issues. However, she was able to validate her areas of emphasis by interviewing several brides to make sure that the subtopics she had identified were inclusive of the wedding experience. Browsing through bookstores to see what couples are buying and reading on their own and reviewing articles in several bridal magazines also identified the skill set that would be needed for this relationship specialty.

Recent journals of family therapy were reviewed for cutting edge research on marriage and couples and for helpful techniques on increased communication skills. Process notes on patients as well as interviews with colleagues who had worked with issues around the planned wedding supplemented the existing materials. Several continuing education workshops presented by the local psychotherapy organization that focused on communication and compromise skills were considered, as well as workshops listed in *The Family Networker,* a professional magazine that focuses on family and couples (see Appendix).

Shaping Your Marketing Materials

The decision was made to "give psychology away" by offering a 2-hour program titled "A Psychological Survival Guide To Your Wedding and Your Marriage" to brides and their grooms. One major marketing consideration was to focus on stores and bridal shops in affluent areas where customers were more likely to seek private practice counseling rather than through a managed care company. In this case, the topic, the evaluation of the marketplace, the skill assessment, and the beginning marketing plan all came together within the first 2 months.

During the 3rd and 4th months, the substance of the talk on wedding survival for brides was developed, along with a flyer that could be distributed at bridal shops. In developing these materials, careful attention was given to the issues that underlie the problems surrounding wedding planning. Because mothers usually accompany daughters for their bridal gown, it was imperative that no statement in the flyer be interpreted whether consciously or unconsciously as threatening to the mother.

Several respected colleagues reviewed the first draft of these materials and provided feedback regarding its content and attractiveness. The flyer was designed on a home computer and photocopied on wedding style paper (lacy design). The flyer in Figure 19.3 is an example of this inexpensive effort.

A PSYCHOLOGICAL SURVIVAL GUIDE TO
YOUR WEDDING
AND YOUR SUCCESSFUL MARRIAGE

FREE 2 HOUR WORKSHOP

Weddings are a symbolic ritual in all societies. Your wedding is significant not just for the day itself, but as a beginning of your marriage. Everyone agrees that wedding days are important to remember, and couples usually spare no expense to make it so.

What will also be very memorable are the psychological moods and interactions between the wedding couple. The psychological mood of the wedding day can and should be planned. To plan this mood, attend a Free 2 Hour Workshop with Psychologist, Dr. Elaine Rodino.

TOPICS TO BE COVERED

* *Communicate, Communicate, Communicate*
* *Basic Values: Similarities and Differences*
* *Your Ideal Wedding: Her Ideal.....His Ideal*
* *Who has more Power? Are you Sure?*
* *Whose wedding is this anyway?*
* *From Wedding Plans to Married Life*

Elaine Rodino, Ph.D. a Licensed Psychologist with more than 20 years experience helping people with relationship issues. She has been quoted on couple issues by newspapers across the country as well as national magazines such as Bride's, Bride Guide, Glamour and McCalls. She is a past president of the Los Angeles County Psychological Association, a Fellow of the Los Angeles Society of Clinical Psychologists, a past president of the Division of Media Psychology, and President-Elect of the Division of Independent Practice of the American Psychological Association.

Elaine Rodino, Ph.D., 1821 Wilshire Blvd., Suite 411, Santa Monica, CA 90403
(310) 828-7772

FIGURE 19.3   Flyer.

Another marketing piece that can be inexpensively produced on your word processor is a fact sheet. You can choose a similar type of "wedding" design paper and color. Remember to include your name, address, phone number, and Web site. Figure 19.4 The following is an example of a fact sheet that can be used for the wedding niche:

Developing Your Networking Contacts and Marketing Distribution Plan

After finalizing these marketing tools, the Yellow Pages was used to generate a list of local bridal shops. The marketing game plan was to ask

FACT SHEET: NINE PSYCHOLOGICAL TASKS NEEDED FOR A GOOD MARRIAGE

- Separate emotionally from the family of one's childhood so as to invest fully in the marriage and, at the same time, to redefine the lines of connection with both families of origin.

- Build togetherness based on mutual identification, shared intimacy and an expanded conscience that includes both partners, while at the same time setting boundaries to protect each partner's autonomy.

- Establish a rich and pleasurable sexual relationship and to protect it from the incursions of the workplace and family obligations.

- For couples with children, absorb the impact of a baby's entrance into the marriage. The couple must learn to continue the work of protecting their own privacy.

- Confront and master the inevitable crises of life.

- Maintain the strength of the marital bond in the face of adversity. The marriage should be a safe haven in which partners are able to express their differences, anger and conflict.

- Use humor and laughter to keep things in perspective and to avoid boredom and isolation.

- Nurture and comfort each other. Satisfy each partner's needs for dependency and offer continuing encouragement and support.

- Keep alive the early romantic, idealized images of falling in love. From the book "The Good Marriage: How and Why Love Lasts" by Judith Wallerstein, Ph.D., 1996, Warner Books.

Adapted from *The Good Marriage: How and Why Love Lasts* by Judith Wallerstein, Ph.D., 1996, Warner Books. Adapted from the tip sheet created by Kelly Cunningham for Psychologists in Independent Practice, a Division of APA.

FIGURE 19.4　A sample fact sheet.

the bridal shop to distribute the announcement. It was anticipated that the bridal shop owners (or department stores) would appreciate the value-added experience because the event would attract customers and increase the likelihood that a gown would be purchased in that shop—clearly a win, win, win situation for the shop, for the practitioner, and for the brides.

The talk would be offered free of charge. However, the therapist would distribute additional materials and be identified and remembered as an expert on marriage and relationships when the new brides considered psychotherapy or marital counseling in the future.

It was planned to offer this program three to four times per year because a one-time event does not create an identify as an expert nor fill a psychotherapist's practice. An evaluation sheet that gets written feedback from the audience can be used to improve your program and for testimonials in future advertising. Be sure to keep a list of the attendees, with their names, addresses, phone numbers, and e-mail addresses so you can let them know of other workshops you may do in the community or have them on a mailing list for fact sheets and articles that you produce in the future. Additional possibilities for advertising this specialty niche include

- distributing flyers in various business locations that would be frequented by brides-to-be, such as florists, pastry shops and bakeries, stationery shops where wedding invitations are purchased.
- contacting wedding planners. Since a more relaxed bride, groom, and mother of the bride are easier clients for wedding planners to work with, these planners may include your flyer with their packet of information to the wedding planning couple.
- discussing a paid newspaper ad placed by the store that will be hosting the workshop. Since the bridal shop will be getting value-added service, they may buy ad space in the local newspaper or even the city's major newspaper to attract customers to their store.
- sending a pitch letter to local newspapers to arouse interest in a story. Invite the reporter to the presentation (this is good marketing for the shop owner as well as for your practice).
- advertising in special bridal brochures that are already left at your local bridal shops.
- creating a 30-minute local access television program on the topic.

As you approach networking contacts with these marketing materials remember that the immediate target group is brides. Typically, brides shop for wedding gowns without their prospective mates. It will most likely be the bride who first becomes aware of the program, and it will most likely be the bride who will convince her fiancé to attend. Once the workshop presentation begins, the long-term target population is the couple.

The wedding niche creates a personal relationship with couples who may someday require psychotherapy. Congratulations! You have carved out a viable, long-term, successful psychotherapy niche.

RELATIONSHIP SUBTOPICS: A MENU OF OPPORTUNITIES

Within the topic of relationships are many marketable niches offering a wide range of exciting practice possibilities. Keep the formula of

Gold Standard Skills + Long Term Marketing = Business Success

in mind as you read each topic below. Consider your personal interests and the professional skills you need to supplement to achieve a gold standard in the subtopics identified in the following.

Couples

Adoption Concerns

Changes in the pattern of adoption have served to increase the need for psychotherapy services. Single men and women and same sex couples are adopting children, raising new questions about childrearing issues and community acceptance. For the prospective adopting parents, the process of adoption is anxiety producing, lengthy, and often filled with apprehension and fear of rejection. Other issues to address include telling children about adoption, deciding if and how to relate to the biological parents, and appreciation and sensitivity to multicultural and racial differences between adopting parents and their children.

Extramarital Affairs

The Clinton and Lewinsky affair had the media in a quest for information about their affair and affairs in general. Separations and divorces may result from an exposed affair, but an affair need not be the end of a marriage. When couples seek psychotherapy and recognize the affair as a problem in the marriage, the relationship can be healed, and the couple then learns to live a more rewarding and fulfilling life together.

Gay and Lesbian Counseling

Although some gay couples and individuals prefer having a psychotherapist who is gay, many either prefer a "straight" therapist or have no preference. To work effectively in this area it is important to understand the intense social differences that occur for gays including discrimination, hate, rejection by family, and the threat and reality of HIV/AIDS.

Postdivorce Counseling

It is sometimes necessary to bring both exspouses into Postdivorce couples counseling in order to successfully execute the court orders for custody and visitation. A specialty in this area is appreciated by attorneys, courts, and schools.

Dual-Career Couple

Adding to the stresses and strains of marriage is the couple who juggles significant career commitments. Careers often compete with the individual needs and are complicated by household, family, and child-rearing responsibilities. In today's work world of virtual technology, both individuals may work from home; at times this can contribute to the existing difficulties.

Family Issues

Family Business

Issues of control, boundaries, guilt, envy, competition, and sibling rivalries are present in this difficult work environment. The family business usually relies on old patterns of behavior that often run counter to good business practices. Birth order and gender issues can undermine business policies.

The Sandwiched Generation

People are living longer, and couples often find themselves "sandwiched" in the middle of two generations who need their help. In addition to the psychological services needed by the suddenly infirm aged parent, the middle generation and the younger generation also require psychological help or at least psychological information. Generational issues can involve control, money, and differences in childrearing ideas. The issue of the sandwich generation spans three generations. Choose your own vantage point, taken from your own accumulated experiences, and decide which group will have your center of focus.

Eldercare

Related to the sandwiched generation, but with a focus on elderly parents and relatives, is the niche of eldercare (Doheny, 2000). By 2002, 42% of workers will be elder caregivers. In a recent study, 22.4% U.S. households included caregivers of people over the age of 50. Seventy-two percent are women, most of whom work outside the home. Eldercare has business opportunities for therapists because lost production due to elder care demands is estimated to be between $11.4 and $29 billion.

Grandparenting

Although being a grandparent is often a joyous event, it can also raise areas of conflict. These areas include grandparents of divorced families, long-distance grandparenting, acceptance of differing childrearing practices, and issues of money and inheritance. In addition, some grandparents are primary caretakers for their grandchildren because of parental death, illness, work needs, or disability. These grandparents often struggle with their own health-related needs as well as the physical, financial, and psychological burdens of childcare.

Health

Infertility

Medical decision making, self-blame, guilt, anger, and financial burdens make this a complex but important niche for clinicians. According to Laurie Kolt,[1] infertility expert, there is some research that indicates "that at the one year mark, women coping with prolonged infertility often had depression and anxiety rates equal to people suffering from life threatening illness, such as cancer or AIDS." Clearly then, the emotional aftermath of infertility lends itself to psychotherapeutic interventions.

Illness

Illness is a family matter. When one person in a family becomes ill, the family equation changes. The needs of the partner, parents, and children are often overlooked as medical and social services are focused on the sick individual. With the aging of the population, health concerns within the context of changing relationships, will be an increasingly marketable niche for psychotherapists.

Disabilities

Disabilities are physical, cognitive, or sensory conditions that limit functioning. Psychotherapists working with such individuals and families focus on issues of exclusion, prejudice, financial hardships, discrimination, and stigma.

Parenting

Shared Parenting

Psychologist Frank Leek[2] has developed what he terms a therapeutic approach to postdivorce coparenting called "Shared Parenting Support Program" (SPSP). He notes that the goals of the program are "to help parents move to the business of co-parenting, form new boundaries after divorce, focus on the needs of the children, undo the child's Paradox (loving two people who are in conflict), reduce parental conflict and provide their children with easy access to each parent."

Single Parenting

The APA (1996) reports that in 1992 single-parent families accounted for 30% of households in the United States, whereas only 25.5% were the traditional two-parent family. Single parenting is an overwhelming responsibility and a very viable niche market issue. Specific issues in the single-parent family can include visitation and custody, continuing conflict between the two biological parents, less time spent with children, the effects of the breakup on the children, their school performance and peer relationships, problems with the extended family relations, issues created by the parents' new dating and new relationships.

Childbirth Adjustment

Couples benefit from assistance in the relationship transition taking place during pregnancy and following the arrival of a first child. Typical concerns include balancing work and family life and resolving differences about topics such as finances, use of babysitters, bedtime and sleeping arrangements, religious practices, and childrearing discipline.

The Difficult Child or Teenager

When there is a difficult child or teen in the family the entire family suffers. Frequently, families deny disruptive behaviors or suffer in silence while enduring major disruptions to their life. Psychotherapists can help parents communicate more effectively with difficult children, can help identify community resources, and can teach positive parenting behaviors. Successfully addressing the issue of difficult children reduces the likelihood of later violence, pregnancy, antisocial behavior, drugs, and suicide.

Learning Disabilities and Attention Deficit Disorder

Psychotherapists can assist with diagnosis and treatment planning for children with learning disorders. Psychotherapists can foster family and school understanding and acceptance of the child with ADHD. By structuring schedules and activities, the therapist can maximize the functioning of the family, minimize the conflicts in the classroom, and enhance the child's self-esteem.

IDENTIFYING YOUR NICHE AND DEVELOPING YOUR PERSONAL MARKETING AGENDA

Earlier in this chapter we supplied ready-made marketing plans focusing on separation and divorce and the wedding niche. In this section, you will identify your professional niche and develop your personal marketing game plan from which you can build a blueprint for success. For the questions below, use some blank paper or start a new file on your computer.

Step 1: Identifying Your Interests

Your specialty niche will need to be an ongoing area of interest and excitement to you. You may already have a specific topic where you enjoy working and simply prefer to further its development. Is there an aspect to your current work that you find intriguing? Which patient problems do you prefer to work with?

If you are looking for a new area of interest, consider your own life circumstances. Your own life experiences and life skills (being multi-lingual, conquering learning problems, becoming an adoptive parent, watching your family struggle with health concerns, participating in a family business) can serve as a springboard for your professional development. List these possibilities here.

As you consider a topic, imagine yourself talking about and working in that area. See if you still like the idea after a few days. Will you enjoy this new niche area? Will it be gratifying and fun and will it fulfill your sense of professionalism?

Step 2: Is Your Niche Viable?

Looking at your responses to step 1, you will want to decide if your topic is a viable niche.

- Is there a consumer need for the services in this niche?
- Are the consumers in your geographical area able to afford these services?
- If consumers are outside the geographical area, are you willing to develop an electronically based practice?
- If consumers are unable to pay for services, are you willing to find agencies to contract with?

Review each of your answers from steps 1 and 2 until you find a niche that both interests you and is viable for the amount and type of marketing you will want to do. Write down your best possibility.

Step 3: The Gold Standard

Are additional skills need to reach the gold standard of skills in this niche? If yes, list the workshops and courses necessary. If you are unsure, list the names of possible mentors that can advise you on a skill-building program.

Step 4: Marketing Materials

What marketing materials do you already have that can be useful in promoting this niche? Will you need to update these materials so that they more clearly identify you as an expert in your niche? Do you need to develop new materials? If so, what types of materials are you most interested in developing. Review the marketing skills chapters and decide on several tools that might be of interest to you.

Step 5: Networking Contacts

All marketing tools need an outlet and will be distributed through individuals that you have some connection with.

- List all marketing efforts you have made in your career, even if you had not previously identified these as "marketing." Include all talks at schools, community, church/synagogue, Kiwanis, and so on.
- List all organizations you participate in, including civic activities, church/synagogue activities, political work.
- List all your networking contacts. Include the obvious professionals who are your colleagues, but also include your own physician, dentist, attorney, as well as others you know in the community.
- List individual neighbors and friends, their occupations and those of their spouses, relatives, or friends they might have mentioned. For example, your neighbor may have mentioned that her sister-in-law is a business executive who could provide a connection for your services.

Step 6: Marketing Distribution Plan

Chapters 11–18 have many suggestions about how to distribute your marketing products. Using your networking list from Step 4, write down to whom you would distribute each of your marketing products. Here are some reminders:

- Business cards—attach these to articles that you distribute at civic activities or groups you attend. Carry them with you at all times because you are bound to be talking to someone about your plans, and you can immediately reinforce the information with a business card.
- Flyers—you can distribute your flyers to individuals who work in or are connected with places appropriate to the topic or issue that you will be marketing. For example, if you are marketing your

work for patients with dental anxiety, distribute your flyers to dentist offices, your local drug store and your physician's office.
- Newsletters—plan a mailing to your old patients and new patients, friends, relatives, and anyone else you know to tell them of a new group or a series of lectures that you will be giving.
- Brochures—brochures can be placed where people usually pick up other brochures. Doctors' offices, divorce attorneys, and the gym.

Be sure to add your Web site and e-mail address to all of your marketing materials and remember to consider using free media exposure as described in chapters 13 and 15.

ESTABLISHING A 6-MONTH TIME LINE: A SAMPLE TO DO LIST

To be successful with your personal agenda, you will need a time line. Remember that there is a big difference between thinking about marketing and doing marketing. Marketing takes discipline and commitment. Your time line schedule needs to be flexible enough to accommodate innovation, research, and feedback but firm enough to discourage procrastination. We recommend setting and writing down specific target dates for each of the steps described in the previous section and holding yourself accountable to these dates.

Months 1 and 2 (Steps 1, 2, and 3)

Schedule time in your weekly calendar for your marketing project. Block out times of the day and week that you will commit to promoting your practice. Honor these times as you would a patient appointment. If you must use the time for some other reason be certain that you "reschedule" that hour or hours just as you would if it were a canceled patient hour that would not be left to the next week. This step is crucial to the success of your project. Consider your target population, where you can access them, who will your referral sources be, what services are already available for this issue, and what services are already available in your area.

Choose your niche area, determine its viability, and investigate the skills you will need to bring you up to the "gold standard." What techniques are other psychotherapists using who work with this issue and how successful have they been? Strengthen your professional skills by reading books, talking to other experts, attending workshops, and checking out the topic on the Web.

Take notes, compile book lists, print out information from Web sites. Is this fun and exciting? If not, perhaps the topic is not one you really want to learn about and use. Think of another "better" topic.

Months 4 and 5

Now that you have decided on your topic, know your population and have strengthened your skills, you are ready to begin to create your marketing approach. If you are planning to develop a workshop presentation or community talk, create this now. Because you will be needing some materials such as brochures, fact sheets and business cards, prepare them now. You will find it helpful to create the materials at the same time you create your talk. Working on one will inspire the other.

Draft and refine each of your marketing products, being sure that whatever you are producing is well-designed. Whether you are working on a brochure, flyer, fact sheet, Web site, or newsletter, be sure that it is attractive, professional, and ethical. Consult someone you respect regarding "the look" as well as the content of the materials. Proofread, proofread, proofread.

Month 6

Take the plunge! You are now ready to get out there and do your stuff. Begin to discuss your ideas and distribute your materials to every potential contact and institution on your networking list. Remember that most people genuinely enjoy being helpful, and you are offering quality services. Most contacts are willing to set up a meeting, recommend your talk, post your flyer, or distribute a brochure. Remember that the media welcomes newcomers, particularly if their information is tied to a community or newsworthy events. Think positive and stay focused on the benefits your service provides.

OUR FINAL WORDS

Marketing consultant Kim Ricketts[3] notes the following:

> As a marketing consultant to mental health professionals, I constantly hear, 'I don't like selling or I don't know how to do marketing.' The message that I like to leave with psychotherapists, psychologists, social workers, etc. is this, The old days of strong arm sales and closing deals' is over. Today, it's all about establishing rapport, listening, resolution and natural conclusion. What professional does all four of these better than

any other professional? Mental health professionals do. The Fortune 500 companies are recognizing this before mental health professionals. Corporate America is hiring psychotherapists to train their marketing and sales staff because they are the experts in the above mentioned areas. When are today's psychotherapists going to reach the same realization?

We hope that you now take on the challenge of achieving an independent psychotherapy practice. You have the ability, the consumer has the need, and professional opportunities are plentiful. Our book helps you surmount the obstacles presented by managed care. *Saying Goodbye to Managed Care* is saying hello to your most creative and professional self. Do what you do best and enjoy your new avenues of professional work.

NOTES

[1] Personal communication, June 10, 1999.
[2] Personal communication, June 16, 1999.
[3] Personal communication, March 3, 1999.

REFERENCES

American Psychological Association. (1996). Family and Relationships: Single Parenting and Today's Family [on-line]. Available: www.apa.org, APA HelpCenter: Get the Facts: Family and Relationships.
Coalition for Marriage Family and Couples Education [on-line]. Available: www.smartmarriages.com, 3/17/00.
Doheny, K. (2000, April). Elder care, younger stress. *Working Woman,* 14.
Faludi, S. (1992). *Backlash: The undeclared war against American women.* New York: Crown Publishers, Inc.
Gottman, J. (1994). *Why marriages succeed or fail and how you can make yours last.* A Fireside Book. New York: Simon and Schuster.

Appendix: Resources

BUSINESS CONSULTANTS

Ackley, Dana, PhD, Psychologist, author, workshop leader, health care practice consultant, business consultant, 3635 Manassas Dr., Ste 1, Roanoke, VA 24018-4053, (540)774-1927, fax (540) 989-8893, danaackley@prodigy.net

Fox, Ronald E., PhD, Psychologist, consultant, American Psychological Association leadership, 104 S. Estes Dr., Ste 301 Chapel Hill, NC 27514-2866, (919) 929-1227, (919) 968-7966 fax (919) 968-2575, email RONALDF625@aol.com, REF@FamilyBusinessDoctor.com, http://www.FamilyBusinessDoctor.com

McGrath, Ellen, PhD, Clinical Psychologist, President and Founder, Bridge Coaching, New York City and Laguna Beach, CA (718) 855-7770, fax (718) 855-1653

Thomas, Mike, PhD, 309 Brookside Drive, Chapel Hill, NC 27516, (919) 781-4343, MCT@FamilyBusinessDoctor.com, www.FamilyBusinessDoctor.com

MEDIA AND MARKETING CONSULTANTS AND INFORMATION

Dick Anderson, Founder and owner: AdVentures, Graphic designer and marketing consultant Creative Consultant for the Family Therapy Networker, 1300 Spring Street, Suite 220, Silver Spring, MD 20910, (301) 495-0484; (800) 262-2221, Fax: (301) 495-0482 advennet@aol.com, http://www.advenweb.com

Bettman Photo Archives. For purchase of stock photos. 902 Broadway, NY, NY, (212) 777-6200

Cunningham, Kelly, Principal ImPRessions, 933 Powhatan Street, Alexandria, Virginia 22314, Office: 703 548-1291, Fax: (703) 548-8090, Cell: 703 855-8211, klcpr@bellatlantic.net

Davenport, Leslie,CSW, Social Worker-psychotherapist. Co director Marketing Advisors for Professionals, New York, NY, (212) 213-9768

Farberman, Rhea—Director Public Affairs, American Psychological Association, 750 First Street N.E., Washington, DC, 20002, (800) 374-2721

Hamlín, Faith—Literary Agent, Sanford J. Greenberger Associates, 55 Fifth Avenue, New York, New York 10003 (212) 206-5607

Kalish, Karen—Media Trainer and consultant, Kalish Communications, 2120 S. Street, NW Washington, DC 20008, (202) 332-3232

Ricketts, Kim, MEd, Strategease Consulting, LLC, P.O. Box 4253, Highland Park, NJ 0809-4253, PH:732-819-0809, Fax: 732-819-0833, email: kimr@ outcomes-dss.com, www.outcomes-dss.com

Steingart, Stacy, Advertising Department, Big Apple Parents Paper, NY, NY (212) 889-6400 x112

PRACTICE BUILDING CONSULTANTS AND AUTHORS

Ackley, Dana. PhD, Psychologist, author, workshop leader, health care practice consultant, business consultant, 3635 Manassas Dr., Ste 1, Roanoke, VA 24018-4053, (540) 774-1927, fax (540) 989-8893, danaackley@prodigy.net

Dean, Ben, PhD, Psychologist/ICF Master Certified Coach, 4400 East West Highway, Suite 1104 Bethesda, MD 20814, (301) 986-5688, fax: (301) 913-9447, ben@mentorcoach.com, www.mentorcoach.com

Haber, Sandra, PhD, Psychologist, author, 1998 President of Psychologists in Independent Practice: a Division of the American Psychological Association, 211 W. 56th Street, Suite 21H, New York, NY 10019, (212) 246-6057, fax (718) 768-4851, email: drshaber@aol.com, www.drhaber.com

Heller, Kalman M., PhD, Psychologist, author, 992 Great Plain Avenue, Needham, MA 02492, (781) 444-3450; fax (781) 449-3134; KHeller714@AOL.com; www.drheller.com

Kolt, Laurie, PhD, Psychologist, author, practice development speaker/coach. Kolt Consulting 1030 Pearl Street, Suite Three, La Jolla CA 92037-1704, (858) 456-2005, fax (858) 592-6080, email—LJKolt@aol.com, website: www.kolt.com

Kovacs, Arthur, PhD Psychologist, Workshop Leader, Futurist, American Psychological Association leadership. 1821 Wilshire Blvd, Suite 411, Santa Monica, CA 90403, (310) 828-4233, fax (310) 828-4992, ALKovacs@aol.com

Lipner, Iris, CSW, BCD, Social worker-psychoanalyst, author, 80 East 11th Street, New York, NY 10003, (212) 353-9721, 808 Carroll Street, Brooklyn, NY 11215, (718) 857-5717, fax (718) 788-8823, email: ILipnerCSW@aol.com, www.IrisLipnerCWS.com

Rodino, Elaine, PhD, Psychologist, author, 2000 President of Psychologists in Independent Practice, a Division of the American Psychological Association. 1821 Wilshire Blvd., Suite 411, Santa Monica, CA 90403, (310) 828-7772, FAX (310) 454-6046, email: ERodino@aol.com, www.DrElaineRodino.com

PROFESSIONAL ASSOCIATIONS

AMHA-NY American Mental Health Alliance-New York. Cooperative of over 250 New York area mental health professionals. (877) AMHANYS, www.AmericanMentalHealth.com

American Mental Health Alliance (877) AMHA007, www.AmericanMentalHealth.com

American Psychological Association—750 First Street, N.E., Washington, DC, 20002-4242, (800) 374-2721

Boulder Psychotherapists Guild (303) 444-1036, www.PsychotherapistGuild.com

Connecticut Psychotherapists Guild (800) 731-8126

Mental Health Cooperative: American Mental Health Alliance-USA, 877AMHA007

National Association of Social Workers, (800) 638-8799, www.socialworkers.org

National Coalition of Mental Health of Mental Health Professionals & Consumers, Inc., (888) SAY NO MC, www.NoManagedCare.org

National Register of Health Service Providers in Psychology—1120 G Street, N.W., Ste 330, Washington, DC, 20005, (202) 783-7663 fax: (202) 347-0550, www.nationalregister.com

New York State Society for Clinical Social Work, Inc., Phone (800) 288-4CSW, www.cswf.org

Psychologists in Independent Practice. A division of The American Psychological Association. Contact: Jeannie Beeaff, (602) 246-6768, email: Div42APA@primenet.com, www.division42.org

PSYCHOTHERAPISTS

Alne, Dennis J., PhD, Psychologist, 2151 E.22nd Street, Brooklyn, NY 11229, (718) 769-4001, ALNED@AOL.COM

Balinth, Noemi PhD,Clinical Psychologist, 110-20 73rd Rd. Suite 2, Forest Hills, NY 11375 Tel. & Fax: (718) 896-5698, DrNoemi@aol.com, http://hometown.aol.com/drnoemi/myhomepage/index.html

Bavonese, Joe, PhD, Psychologist, 123 S. Main Street, Suite 100, Royal Oak, MI 48067, (248) 546-0407, Fax (248) 548-1925, email: drjoe@relationship-institute.com, www.relationship-institute.com

Beer, Lawrence, EdD, Psychologist, Child and Family Psychological Services, P.C., 5380 Holiday Terrace, Kalamazoo, MI 49009, (616) 372-4140, FAX (616) 372-0390, LBBKZOO@AOL.COM, http://members.aol/cfpsinfo/cfps.htm

Bloland, Sue Erickson, CSW, Social worker-psychoanalyst, Co Director Mid Life Mentors, 26 West 9th Street, New York, NY 10011, (212) 982-0275

Brickey, Michael, PhD Psychologist, 865 College Ave, Columbus, OH 43209-2309, (614) 237-5333, fax (614) 237-5333, email: MikeBrickey@att.net, www.DrBrickey.com

Bristol, Judith, CSW, Social worker-psychoanalyst, Co Director Mid Life Mentors, 110-45 71st Street, Forest Hills, NY 11375, Phone (718) 224-8816

Brody, Steve, PhD, Psychologist, author, 4450 Santa Rosa Creek Rd., Cambria, CA 93428, (805) 927-8284, scbrodys@aol.com, www.renewyour-marriage.com

Buckwalter, Jane, CSW, BCD, Social worker-psychoanalyst, President, American Mental Health Alliance New York, 184 Berkeley Place, Brooklyn, NY 11217, Phone/Fax (718) 783-1826

Chang, Alice F., PhD, Psychologist, author, 6616 E. Carondelet Dr., Tucson, AZ 85710-2119, 520-722-4581, email addresses: afchang@azstarnet.com, afchang@cancerhealth.org webpage: www.cancerhealth.org (for the Academy for Cancer Wellness)

Chicurel, Pamela, RN, MS, CS, Clinical Nurse Specialist in psychiatric nursing, 80 East 11th Street, New York, NY 10003, (212) 477-3479.

Cullen, Diana List, CSW, Social worker-psychotherapist, 1999-2000 President, Metropolitian Chapter, New York State Society for Clinical Social Work, 405 East 54th Street, New York, NY 10022, (212) 486-9642 email: Roberta@vny.com

Davenport, Leslie, CSW, Social worker-pychotherapist, Co-director Marketing Advisors for Professionals, New York, NY, (212) 213-9768

Demarais, Ann, PhD First Impressions. 22 Prince Street, Suite 318, NY, NY 10012, (212) 219-0923, email FINYNY@mindspring.com, Interpersonal and self presentation skills

Deitch, Irene, Ph.D, 57 Butterworth, Staten Island, NY 10301-4543, (718) 982-3771 Fax: (718) 273-0990, Deitch@postbox.csi.cuny.edu

Edward, Joyce, CSW, BCD, Social worker-psychoanalyst, 102 Bellhaven Ave, Bellport, NY 11713, (631) 286-3691

Enright, Michael, PhD, Psychologist, P.O. Box 4120, Jackson Hole, WY 83001, (307) 733-7771, fax (307) 733-8276, email: menright@wyoming.com

Fox, Ronald E., PhD, Psychologist, consultant, American Psychological Association leadership, 104 S. Estes Dr., Ste 301 Chapel Hill, NC 27514-2866, (919) 929-1227, (919) 968-7966 fax (919) 968-2575, email RONALDF625@aol.com, REF@FamilyBusinessDoctor.com, http://www. FamilyBusinessDoctor.com

Franklin, Donald, J., PhD, Psychologist, (908) 5526-8111, (908) 806-7344, djfpsych@blast.net, www.psychologyinfo.com/dr_franklin.html

Haber, Sandra, PhD, Psychologist, author, 1998 President of Psychologists in Independent Practice: a Division of the American Psychological Association, 211 W. 56th Street, Suite 21H, New York, NY 10019, (212) 246-6057, fax (718) 768-4851, email: drshaber@aol.com, www.drhaber.com

Harris, Donna, LCSW, Social worker-psychoanalyst. Co-director, New York Association of Trauma. Psychotherapists, 80 East 11th Street, New York, NY 10003, 212 475 4437, 201 837 1619, www.NYAPP.com

Hays, Kate, PhD, Psychologist, The Performing Edge, 730 Yonge Street, Suite 226, Toronto, ON M5T 1M2, Canada, (416) 961-0487, fax (416) 961-5516, email: The_Performing_Edge@compuserve.com

Johnson, Norine, PhD, Psychologist, author, 2001 President of American Psychological Association, 110 W Squantum, #17, Quincy Ma 02171-2122, (617) 471-2268, email: NorineJ@aol.com, www.drnorinejohnson.com

Kilburn Mary, PhD, Psychologist, 4016 Barrett Drive, Suite 104, Raleigh, North Carolina 27609-6623, 919-781-5162 fax 919-781-4754, marykilburn@ mindspring.com, www.mindspring.com/~marykilburn

Kottick, Judith, LCSW, Clinical social worker, Reproductive Medicine Associates of New Jersey, Morristown, NJ, (973) 746-7370

Kovacs, Arthur, PhD Psychologist, Workshop Leader, Futurist, American Psychological Association leadership. 1821 Wilshire Blvd, Suite 411, Santa Monica, CA 90403, (310) 828-4233, fax (310) 828-4992, ALKovacs@aol.com

Lampert, Adrienne, CSW, BCD, Social worker-psychotherapist. 3623 Ave H, Brooklyn, NY 11210, (718) 434-0562, Alamp12619@aol.com

Lavinski, Rosemary, CSW, BCD, Social worker-psychotherapist, career consultant. 868 President Street, Brooklyn, NY 11215, (718) 783-4295, http://members.aol.com/RLavinski

Leek, Frank, PhD, Psychologist, Shared Parenting Support Program, P.O. Box 2468, Fair Oaks, CA 95628, (914) 638-8600, fax (914) 638-8900, SPSP@JSP.net

Lipner, Iris, CSW, BCD, Social worker-psychoanalyst, author, 80 East 11th Street, New York, NY 10003, (212) 353-9721, 808 Carroll Street, Brooklyn, NY 11215, Phone (718) 857-5717, fax (718) 788-8823, email: ILipnerCSW@aol.com, www.IrisLipnerCSW.com

Malin, Leslie, CSW, Psychotherapist, career and life transition coach, Management by Design, Glen Cove, New York (516) 671-5662, www.informeddecisions.com Email: managementbydesign@worldnet.att.net

Marek, Richard, J., LCSW, ACSW, Social worker-psychotherapist, marriage and family therapist, Columbia Commons, 256 Columbia Turnpike, Florham Park, NJ 07932, (973) 377-3600

Massoth, Neil, PhD, Psychologist, 17 Jonquil Ct. Paramus, NJ 07652-1638, (201)444-6253, nmassoth@aol.com

McDermott, Marie, CSW, BCD, Social worker-psychotherapist, 2000 Treasurer, New York State Society for Clinical Social Work, 267 Sixth Ave., Brooklyn, NY 11215, (718) 788-5005.

McGrath, Ellen, PhD, Clinical Psychologist, President and Founder, Bridge Coaching, New York City and Laguna Beach, CA (718) 855-7770, fax (718) 855-1653

Miller, Ivan, PhD, Psychologist, President, Boulder Psychotherapists' Guild, 350 Broadway, Ste 210, Boulder CO 80303-3338, (303) 499-3888, www.PsychotherapistsGuild.com.

Mueller, Janet, PhD, 98-01 67 Ave, Rego Park, New York 11374-4967, (212) 860-5939

Paknis, Gloria T., LCSW, BCD, Social worker-psychotherapist, Director, Solutions for Stress, 37 Kings Road, Madison, New Jersey 07940, 973 377 3966, www.solutionsforstress.net

Perlman, Cheryl, CSW, BCD, Social worker-psychotherapist, 217A Sixth Avenue, Brooklyn, NY 11215, (718) 636-3099.

Phillips, Elizabeth, PhD, LCSW, Past President of the Clinical Social Work Federation, 13 Cooper Rd., North Haven, CT 06473, (203) 248-1510.

Pimental, Patricia, PsyD, ABPN, Board Certified Neuropsychologist; President and CEO Neurobehavioral Medicine Consultants, Ltd., C/O Glenoaks Hospital and Medical Center, 701 Winthrop Ave, Glendale Heights, IL 60139-1405, (630) 856-4632, fax 630-221-8030, dr-patti@interaccess.com

Rios, Susan, CSW, Social worker-psychoanalyst, Co director, New York Association of Trauma. Psychotherapists, 80 East 11th Street, New York, NY 10003, (212) 475-437, www.NYAPP.com

Rodino, Elaine, PhD, Psychologist, author, 2000 President of Psychologists in Independent Practice, a Division of the American Psychological Association. 1821 Wilshire Blvd., Suite 411, Santa Monica, CA 90403, (310) 828-7772, FAX (310) 454-6046, email: ERodino@aol.com, www.DrElaineRodino.com

Sachs, Joyce, PhD, 256 18th St. Santa Monica, CA 90402, (310) 395-6050, fax (310) 556-0832

Schorr, Karyn Figlen, CSW, Social Worker-Psychoatherapist, Co Director Marketing Advisors for Professionals, (212) 213-9768

Shore, Karen, PhD, Psychologist, 1966 Ashley Pl. Westbury, NY 11590-5801 (516) 997-4344, email: kshore@aol.com (or) NCMHPC@aol.com, PO Box 438, Commack, NY 11725

Trachtman, Richard, PhD, CSW, Social Worker-Psychotherapst and Director, MORE Services for MOney & Reltionships, 2166 Broadway, New York, NY 10024, (212) 595-0449, www.moneyandrelationships.com. Email: doctorichard@msn.com

Wachs, Kate, PhD, Psychologist, 875 N. Dearborn, Ste 200, Chicago, IL 60610-3386, (312) 664-4339, fax (312) 337-578, drkate@interaccess.com

Wainrib, Barbara, EdD, Clinical Psychologist,Associate Professor, McGill University, author, 488 Victoria Ave. Westmount, Quebec, Canada H3Y2R4, (514) 481-8272, fax (514) 484-2864, psycrisi@total.net, or psycrisis@aol.com

Walker, Dolores, CSW, JD, Clinical social worker, mediator, attorney, 153 Waverly Place, New York, NY 10014, (212) 691-6073, Dwalkermed@aol.com

Walker, Lenore E., PhD, Psychologist, Walker & Asssociates, Nova Southeastern University Center for Psychological Studies, 3301 College Ave, Ft. Lauderdale, FL 33314, (954) 262-5724, DrLEWalker@aol.com, www.dviworld.org

Williams, Martin, H., PhD,Clinical and Forensic Psychology, P.O. Box 760, Redwood Estates, CA 95044, (888) 225-9957 (voice and fax), Email: mw@drmwilliams.com, www.drmwilliams.com

Wineburgh, Marsha L., CSW, BCD, Social worker-psychotherapist, 263 West End Ave., New York, NY 10025, (212) 595-6518

Zager, Karen, PhD, Psychologist, author, 500A East 87 Street, New York, NY 10128, (212) 628-1768, fax (914) 478-7454, KZager@MINDSPRING.com

Zur, Ofer, PhD, Psychologist, Sonoma Medical Plaza, 181 Andrieux St., #212, Sonoma, CA 95476, (707) 996-0499, FAX: (707) 935-3918, drzur@drzur.com, http://www.drzur.com

WEBSITE CONSULTANTS AND INFORMATION

E-zines: Index to E-zines http://www.e-zine-masterIndex.com; Crash course in publishing e-zines- www.ezineuniversity.com/courses/ez101/101-07sl.htm

Platt, Timothy, PhD, InfoMed Consulting,. Web based information management and consulting, 532 Fourth Street, Brooklyn, NY 11215, (718) 788-7869, infomed_2000@Yahoo.com

Weiss, Rick, Desktop Media of Phoenix, 2808 N 25th Street, Phoenix, AZ 85008, (602) 957-0424, Fax: (602) 957-0499, Rick@desktopmediaphx.com, www.desktopmediaphx.com

WEBSITES FOR HEALTH/MENTAL HEALTH INFORMATION

Coalition for Marriage, Family & Couples Education, 5310 Belt Rd NW, Washington, DC 20015, (202) 362-3332, www.smartmarriages.com Divorce, www.divorcenet.com

Health-Related Sites: www.healthfinder.gov—comprehensive resource filled with links to publications, consumer information and databases, US Dept of Health and Human Services

www.onhealth.com—health and wellness information that is easy to understand.

www.mayohealth.org—medical and health information from the Mayo Clinic.

Imago Institute for Relationship Therapy, www.Imago.com

Mental Health Credentials on line: Metanoia Guide to Internet Mental Health Services—http://www.netabiua.org/imhs/index.html and Internet Mental Health—http://www.mentalhealth.com

National Center for Complementary and Alternative Medicine—PO Box 8218, Silver Springs, MD 20907 (888) 644-6226, fax (301) 495-4957, nccam@altmed-info.org, www.nccam.nih.gov

PsychologistsUSA—free website linkage for licensed psychologists. www.PsychologistsUSA.com. Contact Sandra Haber, PhD, DrSHaber@aolcom or Marty Williams, PhD, mhw@wenet.com

Psychology Information Online, www.Psychologyinfo.com

OTHER

American Psychological Association, Division of Independent Practice. Marketing Brochures, contact 1-877-603-4000

Confertech Bridge Lines. Contact 1-800-252-5150

Dannenberg, Ron—Tax World, 151 7th Avenue, Brooklyn, New York 11215, (718) 857-4300

Farwell, Eric—Mortuary Manager and Past President of the San Diego County Funeral Directors' Association, 611 Momar Lane, Escondido, California 92027 (760) 746-5825, ericf_1998@hotmail.com

Psychotherapy Finances, newsletter published monthly, Phone (561) 624-1155, www.PsychotherapyFinances.com

Visa Credit Card-Contact 1-800-347-8096

Wolf, Elliot—Self Publishing Firm. Elton-Wolf Self Publishers, 2505 2nd Avenue, Suite 515, Seattle, Washington 98121, (888) 281-5965, (206) 748-0345, ewolf@elton-wolf.com

Index

Index